“In this insightful and inspiring story of a [illegible] lam Jarrett provides a primer for how individu[illegible] ould face an unprecedented medical crisis.”



**Dr. John W. [illegible]**
Former Pres[illegible]
Medical Society of New Jersey

“Dr. Adam Jarrett weaves a gripping tale from the front lines of the COVID pandemic and describes how a resilient staff responded without a playbook to care for a tsunami of critically ill patients.”

**Mike Azzara**
Former President and CEO,
The Valley Health Systems

“Dr. Jarrett has been on the frontlines of the Covid-19 pandemic since day one of the outbreak. His first-hand account from initially learning about the virus to landing in the eye of the Covid storm highlights his important role and voice during the pandemic. Dr. Jarrett easily explains the science of Covid, answers our most pressing questions, and educates the reader on simple steps to protect themselves and their family.”

**Josh Gottheimer**
Congressman (NJ-5)

“Holy Name Medical Center was literally ground zero for the pandemic in the U.S. as Covid-19 arrived in the Northeast in March 2020. Dr. Jarrett and his team not only bravely guided their patients and families through an unprecedented time. They were amazing to work with in getting word out to the NYC/NJ community through our daily interviews. This is truly an amazing behind the scenes look at history.”

**Glenn Schuck**
1010 WINS Radio
New York City

# PROLOGUE AND BASIC SCIENCE

It will be helpful for most readers to have a basic understanding of the Covid-19 virus. In the second year of medical school I took a course specifically aimed at teaching us what we needed to know about infectious diseases. I am sure I learned about coronaviruses but, to be honest, I do not recall the specifics of those lessons. If you and I were sitting in that class today the first lesson would go something like this:

Covid-19 is a virus, a form of parasitic life which incorporates into its host's DNA. It hijacks your cells to replicate itself. A perfect virus (from the virus's viewpoint) infects you, but does not kill you; it lives in you and has a long-term relationship with you. The varicella (chickenpox) virus is a good example – it infects you and stays with you forever, sometimes emerging later as shingles. A faulty virus, by comparison, kills the host, and in doing so, kills itself.

Coronaviruses are a family of viruses that are prevalent all around us. It gets its name from the spikes (which are proteins) on its surface that resemble a crown when viewed with a powerful microscope. The spikes on Covid-19 differ from other coronaviruses and probably are what make the virus so dangerous. These spikes enable it to attach to and attack cells, membranes of the nose and lungs, and, in later stages of the infection, even places like the heart muscles.

Coronavirus is one of many viruses that can cause the common cold. (**Covid-19**: **Co** stands for corona, **vi** stands for virus, **d** stands for disease, and the "19" signifies that it was discovered in 2019, not, as some believe, that it is the 19th coronavirus strain – there are seven known strains that infect humans.)

Viruses are always mutating – and successful ones typically mutate in two ways: 1) to become more infectious and more easily spread among humans (as we may have seen with Covid-19), or 2) following the laws of Darwin, to become less deadly – so they do not kill and can live happily ever after in their host.

To the best of our knowledge, the first time a coronavirus crossed over from animals into humans was in 2003, causing Severe Acute Respiratory Syndrome (SARS), which infected approximately 8,400 people and proved fatal for a little more than 11 percent of those infected. The general consensus is that the coronavirus that causes SARS crossed from the palm civet, an animal that most closely resembles a mongoose and is considered a delicacy in some parts of Asia. There have been no known human SARS infections since 2004.

Then, in 2012 another coronavirus crossed from camels to humans, causing Middle East Respiratory Syndrome (MERS). It is likely that eating raw camel meat or drinking camel milk in Saudi Arabia was the cause of the crossover. There has been a total of 2,562 cases worldwide (just two in the U.S)., and over one third of the cases were fatal.

Both SARS and MERS significantly impacted humans, but they were less contagious and did not have the impact that Covid-19 has had on the world.

* * * * *

This story is about my experience as a physician and Chief Medical Officer, and about one hospital's efforts to combat Covid-19. What we did right, what we did wrong, how we used innovation, and the tireless efforts of our entire team.

On Thursday, March 4 of 2020, Holy Name Medical Center evaluated its first patients infected with Covid-19. Thousands of others quickly followed. We were at the epicenter of the first wave to hit the East Coast of America.

This book is not meant to be the definitive authority on Covid-19. Facts evolve, and already I fear that some of the information included here has been surpassed by additional research. However, I believe many of the lessons we learned will apply to future waves of Covid-19 or to the next pandemic. I hope this book can help others and may even help you or the ones you love.

CHAPTER ONE

# It Happened One Morning

*"It will always seem that the best way to address [Covid-19] would be to be doing something that looks like it might be an overreaction. It isn't an overreaction. It's a reaction we feel is commensurate with what is actually going on."*

**Dr. Anthony Fauci**
Director, National Institute of Allergy and Infectious Diseases
March 16, 2020

It was 4:30 a.m., March 16, 2020, and the limo arrived right on time. I had offered to call for an Uber, but I guess CNN's early morning crew had learned from experience that if you want to make sure a guest does not sleep through their alarm and gets to the studio with plenty of time, you send a driver.

The night before, my marketing team had video-linked into my apartment to help me pick out a tie for the interview. I hate ties. I hate the way they feel around my neck. I always have been more comfortable in scrubs. To avoid wearing ties, I often have used the excuse that they are infection magnets. There is clinical evidence that this is true: ties hang loose and can touch patients and their beds. Studies have cultured physicians' ties and they do grow out bacteria. But I could not think of an excuse to not wear one on TV.

After showing my very limited tie collection one by one to the screen, Jessica Griffin of our marketing department (in consultation with my wife, Eileen) picked one that "while not great, will not embarrass the hospital."

I was excited to be on national TV. Early in life I had dreamed of being an actor. Maybe I never gave up the dream. I tried to act nonchalant about the interview with my family – this was really not about my being on national TV, but about educating the public on Covid-19, letting people know about the good work we were doing at Holy Name, and what might be expected for the rest of the country.

It was clear to those of us at Holy Name that this disease was gaining ground – and doing so faster than most people realized. At the time, there were 4,450 cases in the U.S. and 88 deaths (well, at least known deaths). The President had just announced that people traveling from 26 European countries, including Italy, Spain, France, and Germany, would not be allowed into the United States. Holy Name Medical Center was of interest because there were 18 known cases of Covid-19 in Teaneck, the most in any town in New Jersey, and the mayor of Teaneck had just issued an order for a voluntary quarantine.

I had done other interviews in the preceding weeks, but this seemed bigger, and it was the first time that I was doing a joint interview with Holy Name President and CEO Mike Maron. Mike has been with Holy Name for 30 years, working his way up to CFO and then CEO. When the former CEO, Sister Patricia Lynch, was on her deathbed, she grabbed Mike by the collar and said, "Don't screw up my hospital." He takes her charge very seriously.

Mike and I are both bald, middle-aged men. People often remark that we could be related – but he is a much better dresser (he probably picked out his own tie). We may not always agree on everything, but we do agree that Holy Name is a mission-driven hospital that first and foremost cares for its community. Bottom lines are important, but never the most important. Mike is a presence in the room; he speaks forcefully and with conviction. It is easy to see why I was nervous about our first joint appearance. It didn't help that Eileen had texted family and friends to make sure they were awake, alert, and watching.

The ride was uneventful – driving through New York pre-dawn is amazingly quiet and devoid of people. I had no idea that in just a few short weeks, it would be this quiet all day, every day.

In the car, I took time to think about the main points I wanted to make during the 10 minutes we had been told we would be on air:

1. Accurately convey the reality we were seeing at the hospital (a reality not yet fully grasped by the general public, except possibly in Seattle) and our concerns about where the crisis was headed.
2. Explain that we were going to see more cases, but that with aggressive social distancing, we could slow the growth. (I thought I might even explain the realities of exponential growth and how stopping the spread to just one person can have a large impact down the line.)
3. Help put Holy Name on the map as a medium-sized independent hospital that was ahead of the curve handling the caseload of current Covid-19 demands *and* still more than able to handle non-Covid-19 patients.

I arrived at the CNN building in Manhattan around 5:00 a.m. and entered the large reception area, which felt even larger because it was empty, save for a single guard. No signs yet of social distancing, hand sanitizers, or face masks. The guard directed me to the elevator and up I went, unescorted, to the green room, where guests wait before going on air.

The hall to the green room was lined with posters of Anderson Cooper, Christiane Amanpour, and Chris Cuomo looking down on you – I found it a little reassuring, but at the same time a little intimidating.

When I arrived at the green room, I discovered that this one was not green. It was longer than it was wide, with a window overlooking Manhattan. There were high-top chairs and a couch – no food or coffee. (I had been expecting at least a bagel or two.) In one of the chairs sat Mike and, in the other, a child psychiatrist who was going on before us to discuss how to talk to your children about Covid-19. She was from Cornell University Medical Center New York Hospital, where I had trained, and we briefly talked about our times there while my boss texted with an employee in public affairs.

The child psychiatrist was escorted out to the studio, and we watched her segment on a large screen television in the room. She did well. She later became a regular, discussing psychiatric issues and Covid-19 on the CNN morning show, though for her future segments she was interviewed remotely.

As her segment finished, a technician wired us with mics and earpieces so we could hear what was live.

On the sound stage, Mike and I were seated at two adjacent chairs in a staged living room, with an empty chair for the anchor. It was one of three sets, all positioned in the one studio.

As the two anchors went to a break, we situated ourselves. The male anchor grabbed his papers and ran out; Alisyn Camerota, the other anchor, came over and greeted us. "He wants to be nowhere near you two," she said with a chuckle. I was a little taken aback, but then thought to myself that I was likely going to hear this many more times in the ensuing months (maybe even from family) – and asked myself: could I blame them?

When the cameras turned on, Alisyn jumped right in. "You have a colleague in critical condition. What can you tell us about him?"

My mind went immediately to one of our staff, a worker in food services who was in the Intensive Care Unit (ICU). He was not doing well. He was well-known and well-loved at the hospital and his coming down with Covid-19 had had a noticeable impact on the atmosphere at the hospital. People were realizing, "This could happen to me."

I answered, "We've had several staff members who developed coronavirus because of a community-acquired case and one of them is critically ill in the ICU." Not stated very eloquently, but I was thrown off that this was the first question and was not sure whether I should have let Mike answer it.

In all, the interview lasted four and a half minutes. After it was over, the crew pulled off our microphones and earpieces and Mike and I took a quick photo at the anchor desk, with Alisyn between us. We were then sent on our way.

Leaving the studio, both Mike and I were disappointed. We felt we had failed to cover the critical issues. While Mike and I were (somewhat naively) interested in educating the public and making them feel the reality of what was happening on the frontlines, CNN had grabbed hold of what felt like a public interest story.

Mike and I shared the backseat of the CNN car on the drive to the hospital to start our workday – still early, so without traffic. The normally 30- to 40-minute ride took just 20 minutes.

The ride was mostly quiet. I worried that I had spoken too much (which I have been told I do on occasion) and I was concerned with how Mike might react. And I was disappointed in my delivery. I hate when I stumble on my words, which I felt I had. I had done several interviews in the preceding weeks on NJTV with a great reporter, Michael Hill (who later took time off because his mother died of Covid-19), as well as regular interviews with Glenn Schuck of 1010 WINS a New York City all-news station. (Glenn and I had hit it off instantly – in part because I had been his father's doctor when I was in private practice.) I had thought I was getting good at this, that I was ready for the big leagues.

I spoke first. "I think I stepped on some of your answers and it may have come across as us not being as confident as we needed to be." Mike seemed to shrug this off, but replied, “If we do more interviews together, we need a game plan for who is going to handle which questions.” If he had concerns beyond that, he did not let me know.

Despite our own critical view of the interview, we received positive comments from co-workers and family throughout the day. I even heard from some medical school classmates for the first time in decades.

I spent a fair amount of time with Mike that day, not to mention all the time we had spent together in preceding days:

- Twenty minutes on the same couch in the green room.
- On stage for five minutes in adjacent chairs.
- Standing close together for the picture at the CNN anchor desk.
- Twenty minutes sharing the backseat of the car to Holy Name.
- Attending several meetings throughout the day.

Two days later, Mike, his wife, and his son were diagnosed with Covid-19. He had been in the early, and infectious, stage of the virus the entire day of the CNN interview.

Mike and I on the set of CNN with Alisyn Camerota. No face masks and no social distancing.

**On March 16, 2020**

- 167,515 people worldwide have been diagnosed with Covid-19, with 6,606 deaths.
- For the first time, there are more cases outside of China than inside.
- Canada places restrictions on non-citizens crossing the U.S.-Canada border.
- WrestleMania 36 plays before an empty arena in Orlando, Florida.

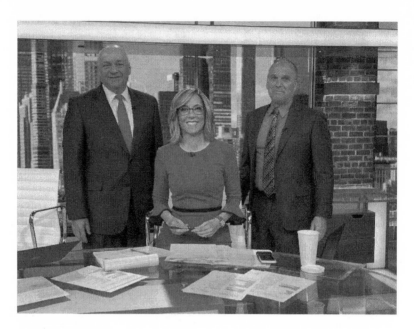

CHAPTER TWO

# It Arrives on Our Shores

*"It was scary, because every morning when you got up, you asked, 'Who died during the night?' You know death was there all the time. People were very leery of each other. And when we went out, we wore a mask over our noses and mouths."*

**Kenneth Crotty**
Remembering his time as an 11-year-old boy during the Spanish flu
2005

Sitting on a New Jersey beach, you often do not even notice the tide is coming in until a big wave overwhelms you and your towel – Covid-19 was like that. But then there was a bigger wave and a bigger wave. And each day, you thought you and everyone around you would be consumed. After weeks and months of daily bigger waves, they subsided, but every day you wondered whether another wave would come – and if it would be bigger still. We never knew whether the force of the wave would knock us down, drag us under, and leave us gasping for air – much like many of our Covid-19 patients – or if we could stand strong and maintain our footing, bracing for the inevitable next wave.

* * * * *

At Holy Name, we had been tracking the advance of Covid-19 in China, France, and Italy pretty closely for several months. When cases popped up in Washington State, New York City, and just over the New York-New Jersey border in the Orthodox Jewish community of Westchester, New York, we knew that it would not be long before a Covid-19 patient would come through our emergency room doors.

On Wednesday, March 4 at 2:23 p.m., Mr. Perez, an obese 45-year-old Hispanic male who was otherwise healthy, with the exception of high blood pressure, came to our Emergency Department (ED, the new term for emergency room).

He had been sick for one week with a cough and fever. He had not traveled recently and had not been in contact with anyone else who had been ill, but he had a chest X-ray that was consistent with Covid-19 pneumonia. Despite his lack of travel, we were concerned that he might be our first case. We prescribed antibiotics, gave him intravenous (IV) fluids, and put him on oxygen.

Mr. Perez was not the only one. On that day, we admitted six patients with Covid-19 to Holy Name. By the end of that weekend, we had 13, including one who went directly onto a ventilator.

By Monday, we knew we were in a crisis and it was all hands on deck. We were off and running, desperately trying to keep ahead of the demands on the hospital – the needs for specialized negative pressure rooms (critical for infectious patients), medical and personal protective equipment (PPE), adequate supplies of medications, and the absolute necessity of maintaining an adequate and healthy staff.

Five days later, we had 32 suspected patients (though no lab-confirmed cases yet) likely sick with this highly infectious disease that we knew very little about – a disease with no proven treatments, with more patients arriving every hour.

Mr. Perez continued to worsen and was placed on a ventilator. By that point, most of us were convinced he had Covid-19, as most young healthy patients with pneumonia just did not get this sick. Ten days into his admission, I received a call from the head of Infection Control. "Adam, Mr. Perez is our first confirmed case...."

Any doubt that remained was gone; it was here. I sat back in my chair, took a deep breath, closed my eyes for a brief moment, and then got back to work.

When I went home that night, I climbed into bed with Eileen, exhausted, and for the first time wept, really wept. I wept because I feared that we might not be able to keep up, that we might end up having to compromise care, and that many patients and families were going to suffer. And I knew that some of my co-workers, people I knew and truly cared for, were likely going to die. Eileen hadn't seen me break down like this since my first week on a New York City AIDS ward over thirty years earlier. She knew that the situation at the hospital was serious and getting worse.

That night, despite my fatigue, I slept fitfully, thinking about the possibility of hospital hallways lined with stretchers filled with suffering patients not being cared for – not just because of a dramatic increase in patients, but because the staff itself could be decimated by the virus. Over the next few days, Mr. Perez continued to worsen. He went into kidney failure and died shortly after.

The situation was emotionally overwhelming for everyone at the hospital. Within days of our first Covid-19 case, the feared code blue (cardiac arrest) message over the loudspeaker had changed from an occasional occurrence to a steady reminder of how bad the situation had become – and the number of people walking through the doors of our hospital seeking care was steadily growing. It was clear that people – many people – were going to die. As a physician, I was prepared for these realities; it was the nature of healthcare and, more frighteningly, the nature of this specific virus.

* * * * *

I started my career as an internal medicine physician in Bergen County, New Jersey. In 2005, after practicing medicine for 13 years and recently graduating from NYU's Healthcare Administration master's program, I became the Chief Medical Officer (CMO) of a 115-bed hospital in Northern New York. After five years of learning how to run a small, rural organization, I was ready to move on to a bigger challenge. In 2010, I became the CMO of Holy Name Medical Center, a 360-bed hospital in Teaneck, New Jersey. Although I didn't know much about Holy Name's history when I started, I was thrilled to be back in Bergen County, and I was impressed with Mike and the rest of the Holy Name staff. As I learned more about the hospital's story during my first few months on the job, I became convinced that I had landed in the right spot.

Holy Name Medical Center sits on a hill just off Route 4 in Teaneck, New Jersey, a short drive from the George Washington Bridge. Holy Name Hospital (as it was called until 2010 and is still referred to by many) was founded seven years after the Spanish flu pandemic, which ravaged the country in 1918 and 1919. Following closely on the heels of World War I, the Spanish flu infected 500 million people worldwide and caused 50 million deaths. It spread around the globe more slowly than Covid-19; we were a less mobile society then, and the Spanish flu came to the U.S. with the return of soldiers from the war. In the U.S., approximately 675,000 people died, more than during the Civil War. Unlike the typical flu, the Spanish flu was unique in that it killed otherwise healthy people, with three age groups hit particularly hard: those under five, those over 65 and, and unusually, those 20 to 35.

Although no one knows for sure, there are various theories that might explain why there was such a high mortality rate among the 20 to 35 age group:

1. The older population had developed some immunity during an earlier flu outbreak before the younger generation was born.
2. Twenty- to 35-year-olds had higher rates of tuberculosis (TB), which caused higher mortality in combination with Spanish flu.

3. Twenty- to 35-year-olds may have had an overactive immune response compared to the older population. (This may be similar to responses to Covid-19 in young people.)
4. Those who were 20 to 35 during the Spanish flu had been the most at-risk age group when they were children during the Russian flu of 1889-1890. That earlier flu may have caused an abnormality in the immune system that made those patients more susceptible to secondary bacterial pneumonia when they contracted the Spanish flu.

The Spanish flu devastated the U.S., but it affected different areas of the country in different ways depending on the responses of local officials and the safeguards those officials put in place – or failed to put in place.

For example, St. Louis, Missouri, took early action. Officials closed schools and places of public gathering and the city had a vocal public health leader advocating for the necessary steps to minimize spread. As a result, St. Louis successfully stemmed the tide of Spanish flu cases.

Philadelphia's public health director, in contrast, downplayed the virus. He told the citizens of Philadelphia that the virus infecting returning soldiers stationed at the Philadelphia Navy Yard would not impact non-military citizens. Even once the Spanish flu began to spread outside the military, he ignored the risk. Rather than shut down the city, he kept businesses open as usual and insisted on holding a planned parade – one of the first recorded super-spreader events, with over 200,000 people in attendance. One week after the parade, the city's hospitals were full, and the death count had reached 4,500. The final toll in Philadelphia: 500,000 infected and 14,000 dead. During the first six months of the pandemic, Philadelphia had twice as many Spanish flu deaths per 100,000 people as St. Louis.

Of course, doctors in 1918 did not have the medicines and healthcare services we have today. If they had, perhaps many of the Spanish flu deaths could have been prevented. But even today, we cannot provide care to every Covid-19 patient if our hospitals reach capacity. This makes the goal of slowing down the spread of Covid-19 essential. The supportive medical care and experimental treatment we have today has the potential to save lives – if our system is not overwhelmed.

After the Spanish flu, the fear that existing medical facilities would be woefully inadequate to deal with another pandemic prompted New Jersey doctors Frank McCormack and George Pitkin to advocate for a new hospital in growing Bergen County. In 1925, the doctors approached Mother General Agatha Brown of the Sisters of St. Joseph of Peace order, who promptly arranged to purchase a site for the new hospital.

When Holy Name's first patient arrived in 1925, the facility had 115 beds, fewer than a dozen physicians, and nurses who, for the most part, were members of the Sisters of St. Joseph of Peace. Today, the Holy Name medical system has 361 beds and a medical staff of more than 1,000 doctors. The medical staff is aided by more than 3,900 employees at approximately 80 different locations affiliated with Holy Name.

Just under 100 years after its start, and a little later than they probably expected, the hospital founded by Drs. McCormack and Pitkin and Mother Brown was called into action to fulfill its original purpose – responding to a pandemic.

**On March 27, 2020**

- The U.S. has more than 101,000 Covid-19 cases, becoming the country with the most cases in the world.
- The U.S. passes a historic $2 trillion stimulus package to counter Covid-19's economic impact.
- The state of Arkansas requests that anyone traveling into the state from New York self-quarantine for fourteen days.
- In Italy, a 102-year-old woman is discharged from a hospital after a 20-day admission for Covid-19. Her doctors hypothesize she might be the first patient to survive both Covid-19 and the Spanish flu and collect serum samples for further study.

CHAPTER THREE

# Our Early Patients

*"We're trying to keep our heads above water without drowning. We are scared. We're trying to fight for everyone else's life, but we also fight for our lives as well."*

**Dr. Arabia Mollette**
Emergency Medicine Physician, Brooklyn, New York
March 31, 2020

When the first Covid-19 patients arrived at Holy Name, we thought we were prepared. We had met regularly to discuss news from China, then Italy and Spain. We had run through scenarios and what-ifs, and we had a plan. We thought it was a good one.

The plan incorporated key lessons from two other threats we had faced: severe acute respiratory syndrome (SARS) and Ebolavirus (Ebola). In 2003, Holy Name had successfully treated the first SARS patient in the United States, a pregnant woman who later delivered a healthy baby girl despite her illness.

Ebola emerged in West Africa in 2014 and created a mild panic in the U.S. When I first heard of Ebola, I thought, "Could this be the next Spanish flu?" It was one of those dreaded diseases you read about but hoped never to encounter, like the bubonic plague. Ebola ultimately killed more than 11,000 West Africans, and there are still sporadic cases in Africa today. In the U.S., we had 11 cases, seven of who were infected outside the country. Two of those patients died, but we haven't had a case in the United States since 2014.

Because the expected threats of SARS and Ebola never materialized in the U.S., they may have lulled us – and the whole nation – into thinking it was prudent to plan, but not to worry. A full-blown pandemic couldn't happen here.

Before we admitted our first Covid-19 patients, the heart of Holy Name's strategy had been to keep those patients, and the staff who cared for them, separate from the rest of the medical center's operations – starting from the moment the patients arrived. Our plan centered on the ED. These emergency departments are no longer one large room, but rather whole wings of hospitals with their own very specialized equipment and staff. To keep Covid-19 patients separate, we partitioned our ED to dedicate a portion of it to the diagnosis and care of Covid-19 patients.

By placing Covid-19 patients in the separate Covid-19 "emergency wing" within the ED, we would eliminate the need to move contagious patients from the ED to elsewhere in the hospital, decreasing the risk of spreading the disease. However, this would take up ED beds that would normally be free for other patients, creating longer waits for run-of-the-mill athletic injuries, garden mishaps, or other conditions that may require hospitalization.

This was a shift for Holy Name. We strive to avoid long waits in the waiting room and once patients are transferred to an ED bed, we aim to quickly shift them to specialized floors or wings when needed. We hoped most patients who experienced waits in the ED as a result of Covid-19 would understand that we had to reallocate resources to ensure their safety, but it did feel as if we were compromising care for the non-Covid-19 patients – which was not ideal.

To prepare, at the end of February, we equipped and isolated six beds in the ED (one-eighth of our ED total) for Covid-19 patients. We created negative pressure rooms, identified the key staff who would care for the patients located in them, and ran simulations to make sure we were ready.

These negative pressure isolation rooms were a key component of our plan. Negative pressure rooms are designed to protect those outside of the room. Fans continually suck air, and any virus suspended in it, out of the room and force it through filters. These filters trap the virus before releasing the virus-free air into the general environment.

Negative pressure rooms are especially important when a virus is spread by aerosol, small portions of the virus that can remain in the air. Aerosolized viruses can also get deeper into the lungs more easily, causing lower respiratory infection. Covid-19 likely spreads by both aerosol and droplets – and may spread differently in different settings. In the hospital, we needed to take precautions against aerosolized transmission of the virus to avoid infecting more patients, as well as staff.

Typically, every hospital has a few negative pressure rooms. These rooms are mainly used to treat patients with airborne infections such as TB. TB is not as contagious as Covid-19 (at least not in the U.S.), but its impact on patients is severe, and treatment has become increasingly difficult as TB has become more and more resistant to drug treatment. TB also has a longer incubation period than Covid-19 – a person who contracts TB might not show any symptoms for years. When I dealt with TB in residency, hospitals were not yet consistently using negative pressure rooms; some physicians were not even familiar with the concept. In fact, the Center for Disease Control (CDC) didn't develop its first set of formal guidelines for negative pressure rooms for the treatment of TB and other diseases until 2003. Looking back, I am amazed that more healthcare workers did not get TB. Today, I definitely would not want to care for active TB patients without negative pressure rooms.

The Covid-19 beds in Holy Name's ED quickly filled. It became obvious that we had drastically underestimated the number of Covid-19 patients who would require treatment (both those who would receive out-patient treatment and those who would require hospitalization) and how long this crisis would last. In retrospect, it is hard to believe that we had thought this would be a short-term problem that we could handle with only six beds in the ED.

On Wednesday, March 11, just a week after we had admitted our first Covid-19 patient (or our first *known* Covid-19 patient), we realized that six Covid-19 beds would not be enough. We began to expand our Covid-19 ward in the ED: first, nine more beds on that Wednesday, then five more on Thursday and four more on Friday. By this time, half of the ED was dedicated to Covid-19 patients – a total of 24 beds. We ended each day thinking, "We dodged a bullet, but we're fine." But each morning, we would scramble to meet the needs of even more Covid-19 patients – an increasing number of who were in critical condition.

As the flow of Covid-19 patients steadily grew, it became clear that isolating Covid-19 patients in the ED was not going to be enough. We needed to take more dramatic action. By March 13, we had added Covid-19 beds on a medical floor, creating an additional 10 negative pressure rooms for non-critical Covid-19 patients. The demand for intensive care beds continued to rise, however, and very quickly outstripped the capacity of our ED. On March 14, we added six Covid-19 beds to our regular ICU – then added 10 more Covid-19 ICU beds a few days later.

When you think of hospital workers, you might think of nurses, doctors, and maybe a friendly receptionist who greets you at the front desk. You probably do not think of facility workers and engineers, employees who design and build. But these people are critical to the working of a hospital – especially in times of rapid-fire challenges, both large and small.

Each time we expanded our Covid-19 facilities to new areas of the hospital, these workers constructed walls, installed vents, and made the other changes necessary to enable us to care for Covid-19 patients. Most notably, this team converted ordinary patient rooms to negative pressure spaces – and they got quite good at it.

The crew started this process by knocking out a room's window and covering it with plywood. They then attached an HVAC (heating ventilation and air conditioning) duct to the window and ran the duct up the side of the building to the roof, where they connected it to a high-powered fan. That fan pulled the air from the room (including any aerosolized virus) up through filters – filters that the facilities team would later clean while decked in full hazmat gear.

At the height of Covid-19, the many ducts leading from rooms to roof made Holy Name look like a giant spaceship with tentacle-like landing gear easing down onto the hospital grounds. The steady flow of air out of a room through this specialized ductwork was critical to stopping the virus from spreading to other parts of the hospital.

Years ago, auditors would test the efficacy of negative pressure rooms by dropping a sheet of paper on the floor outside the closed door. If the paper was whisked into the room, the auditor knew that air was flowing from the hallway into the room and that potentially dangerous air was not escaping back into the hospital through the door. Even when the door of a negative pressure room is opened all the way, air continues to flow into the room rather than out, keeping any virus contained. Today, each room has a gauge and alarms to monitor the pressure and alert the staff if the air begins to flow out of the room (although some old-school inspectors still like the paper test). However, during Covid-19, there was no time to set up the gauges and alarms – even if enough could have been found to meet the surging need.

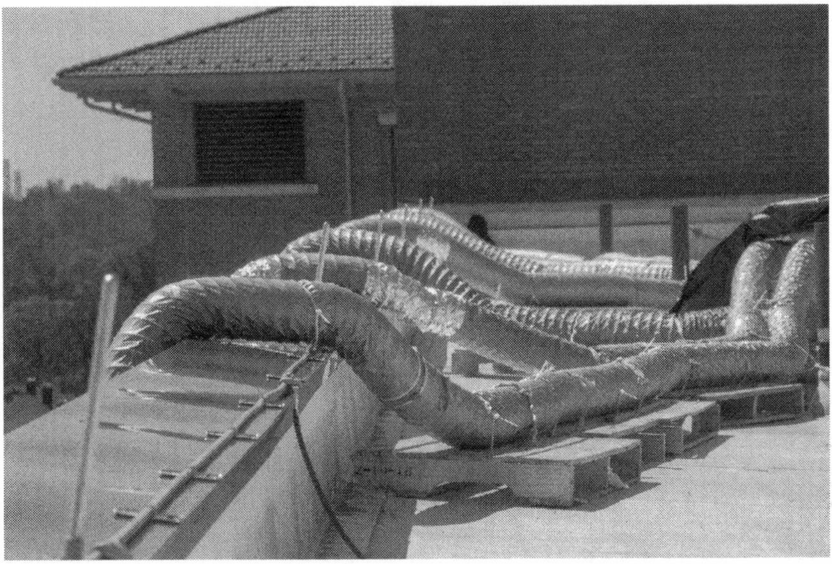

HVAC ducts draped off the roof of the hospital running down to negative pressure rooms.

Our facilities team decided to remove the doors to each room, then duct tape plastic tarps across the entryways and place zippers down the middle. Each doorway looked like the entrance to a camping tent, but the plastic sheets in the hospital kept the aerosolized virus in, rather than keeping mosquitos out. The concave curve of the plastic let us easily monitor the rooms and know that the negative pressure was working correctly. The clear plastic also meant that nurses and doctors could see patients without going in and out of the rooms, which minimized the need to change PPE.

In the early days of the pandemic, both the CDC and the New Jersey Department of Health recommended the use of negative pressure rooms for testing and treatment of suspected Covid-19 patients. Testing requires swabbing high into the nasal passage, which often triggers sneezing or coughing. If the testee is contagious, this sends out a gush of virus, endangering anyone in the vicinity (this is why hospitals and testing centers across the country often tested patients outside in open air with staff in full PPE). In negative pressure rooms, any virus expelled during testing would be quickly sucked into a filter.

At Holy Name, we quickly committed to treating all Covid-19 patients in negative pressure rooms and created a testing site outside so we could safely swab a high volume of patients.

One evening about two months into the pandemic, I turned on the television to see a news conference with New York Governor Andrew Cuomo about the importance of testing. Cuomo wanted the audience to see in real time how easy it was to get tested. Out came a healthcare worker in full PPE, who proceeded to perform a nasopharyngeal swab on the Governor. Cuomo tolerated the procedure well; most patients reflexively pull back from the swab, but he did not. I was astonished, however, that the swab was not done outside, nor in a negative pressure room. I found it hard to believe that the Governor and New York State healthcare officials would blatantly disregard formal CDC recommendations, even – or perhaps especially – on live TV.

As I watched, I pulled out my laptop and went to the CDC website. To my surprise, the guideline had changed. The CDC no longer recommended negative pressure for the testing or treatment of Covid-19 patients. This made no sense to me. Maybe there was some doubt as to whether the virus was aerosolized, but the virus was too deadly to take any chances. How could we put our healthcare workers at risk?

Since then, the CDC has partially reverted its position. Its current stance (as of October 5, 2020, its most recent update on this issue) is that the transmission of Covid-19 typically occurs via droplets but can also, under certain conditions, occur via aerosols. Those conditions include being in enclosed spaces with infected individuals, having prolonged exposure to respiratory particles, and being in a room with inadequate ventilation. Each of those conditions occur in hospitals when patients are cared for outside of negative pressure rooms. So why has the CDC not returned to its position requiring the use of negative pressure rooms? I don't know for sure but, I have a few thoughts.

Is the CDC concerned that hospitals cannot meet the logistical demands of creating adequate numbers of these rooms? Has it received governmental pressure to not take a strong stand on this issue? Or has it decided that the science is too inconclusive to provide definitive guidance?

I am not sure we will ever fully understand the CDCs motivations, but I am fully convinced that negative pressure is essential when testing and treating Covid-19 patients. Our healthcare workers are our most valuable resource, and keeping them safe is not only critical to ensuring that we can provide the highest quality care to our patients, but also our moral obligation.

Three weeks after our first patient arrived, our admitted Covid-19 patient count reached, and then, exceeded 100. The population of Covid-19 patients coming to the hospital was incredibly diverse: all ages (except pediatrics) and all ethnicities (though over time, we saw more and more people of color). We seemed to be seeing slightly more men than women, and it was clear early on that patients who were overweight – even slightly – were getting more severely ill than those who were not. Most patients had no significant travel history and, frighteningly, many patients had no known exposure to Covid-19. Clearly, the disease was running rampant in the community. Any previous thought that we need only be concerned about patients traveling from Asia or other places outside of the U.S. was just completely wrong.

In addition to a growing number of admitted patients, we were also seeing a rapidly increasing volume of patients that did not require hospitalization, but did require careful outpatient follow-up. By mid-March, many local physicians' offices had closed, and symptomatic patients were being instructed to go directly to the hospital to avoid further spreading the virus. As a result, patients who would have received care for an illness like Covid-19 in their doctors' offices were instead arriving at the ED, adding to the already staggering number of patients we were treating. By the end of the first wave of the pandemic, we had managed well over 7,000 Covid-19 outpatients. Many of these patients just needed a phone call every few days and reassurance that their condition was stable. A smaller population needed more intensive telemedicine with at-home monitoring of vital signs and oxygen levels. And an even smaller subset of patients deteriorated and ultimately required hospitalization.

As the number of admitted patients increased, the number of patients dying rose as well. Staff was exhausted, with many working long shifts with no days off. And we were constantly concerned that we would run out of negative pressure rooms, a situation that would put both patients and staff at risk. Covid-19 care took over the entire pediatric and adult medicine wards, as we converted those rooms to negative pressure. In the preceding weeks, these wards had emptied as patients stopped coming in for elective surgeries. Others who desperately needed treatment chose to stay home – even when a hospital visit might have saved their lives.

This was the unfortunate case with the father-in-law of one of our physician network administrators, Jill Hurley. Jill's father-in-law had been feeling poorly for about a week. Partially related to his stoicism, but also because of Covid-19, he hesitated to come to the hospital. He was tired and had severe indigestion on and off, then on the tenth day of his illness, he began to cough and couldn't catch his breath. The family, convinced that Mr. Hurley had Covid-19, took him to our ED. His Covid-19 test came back negative. The family and I were relieved, but we were also very concerned.

Mr. Hurley had a fever, low oxygen levels, and a chest X-ray consistent with heart failure. His EKG showed he had suffered a heart attack, probably about 10 days earlier. He continued to have insufficient blood flow to his heart, so we brought him to the catheterization lab, where our team could evaluate any abnormalities in his coronary artery anatomy. Mr. Hurley not only had significant blockages of his arteries, but also a hole in the septal wall of his heart – a critical condition that needed immediate intervention. In the lab, our staff inserted an intra-aortic balloon pump into his groin and guided it into his aorta so it could help his heart pump. The goal was to stabilize him so that he could undergo open-heart surgery.

Mr. Hurley, like all our patients during Covid-19, went through all of this with no family at his side. One of our anesthesiologists who knew Jill quite well spoke with him in a reassuring manner, stroked his forehead, and told him how much his family loved him. Mr. Hurley kept thanking her.

Unfortunately, Mr. Hurley had also contracted pneumonia and never was well enough for the surgery to be performed. As he began to decline further, based on wishes that he had previously expressed, the Hurley family made the difficult decision to withdraw care and let him die in peace.

There is no way to know for sure, but it is extremely likely that if Mr. Hurley had come in earlier, we could have saved his life – and we also could have protected him from Covid-19. Early treatment of heart attacks has all but eliminated the complications he suffered: septal wall rupture, heart failure, and pneumonia.

While Mr. Hurley's death was not categorized as a Covid-19 death, he likely would not have died but for the Covid-19 crisis. And he was not the only one. We will never know how many people died this type of "non-Covid-19 Covid-19" death, but my guess is that it is a significant number. This number includes not just those who had heart attacks and strokes and put off going to the hospital until it was too late, but also people who put off routine visits – visits that may have caught skin, ovarian, or other cancers early on, when they could most successfully have been treated.

While the hospital saw a drop in these routine appointments, some non-Covid-19 wards were still busy – for instance, babies kept coming. Maternity wards presented several challenges during Covid-19. While we did not know for certain early on if pregnant mothers who had Covid-19 could pass it on to their children before birth or during delivery, the initial evidence suggested that they did not. There now seems to have been a handful of cases where there was "vertical transmission" from mother to baby, although the science on this is not yet definitive. However, we did know that a mother with Covid-19 could infect a baby once born.

This caused a debate amongst medical staff as to whether we should test every expectant mother. The anesthesiologists, who are physically closest to a patient's airway during delivery, argued yes. Obstetrics and nursing staff argued no; they didn't want to separate mothers and newborn babies. The first few days after birth are a crucial bonding time for both the mother and the baby and can have a huge impact on a child's development. Initially, I sided with those who said no, and we only tested pregnant patients who had symptoms of Covid-19 or who had been exposed to the virus. Aside from the psychological impact of separating parents and newborns, we had a shortage of tests, and it took so long for results to come back that they were often irrelevant by the time we received them.

Information coming out of New York Presbyterian Medical Center, however, showed that there were expectant mothers who were Covid-19-positive but asymptomatic. Were we putting the soon-to-be-born babies at risk? We changed our policy and began to test every pregnant patient – and found several who were positive and asymptomatic. All staff were already wearing full PPE when interacting with patients, so we did not need to make any operational changes. However, if a mother had Covid-19, she could not interact with or hold her child during the critical first two weeks of life – a heart-wrenching situation.

One excited couple was expecting their first baby. After several early pregnancy miscarriages, they were naturally on edge, even before Covid-19 hit. Once it did, they stayed in close contact with their obstetrician and limited their contact with the "outside world." Neither future parent had any symptoms of Covid-19. They were sure they were safe from the virus and its possible impact on their baby.

By the time they arrived at Holy Name in the early stages of labor, we were testing all expectant moms. The mother-to-be's test came back positive. They were shocked. Could the test be wrong? It did not matter. We had to assume she was positive and that any contact with the baby after delivery might be dangerous. We explained this to the parents, who understood, but were understandably and visibly upset.

Their baby girl was delivered four hours later, with the entire staff and the father gowned in full PPE. Immediately after the delivery, without any chance for the new parents to bond with their daughter, baby Sara was quickly taken from the delivery room to an isolation nursery, where she was Covid-19 tested – and thankfully received a negative result.

The parents were devastated to be separated from their baby (because the father had been exposed to Covid-19 through his wife, there was a risk he also could transmit the disease), but they understood. The entire obstetrics team was upset as well. But at the time, we did not see any other alternative.

Several weeks later, the American College of Gynecology came out with a formal statement: it recommended that newborn babies of Covid-19-positive moms have protected contact with their parents, and even encouraged allowing the baby to remain in the room with the new mother.

This was a controversial recommendation, but clearly was motivated by concern for the psychological impact of early separation. We responded to this recommendation by sharing it with parents and allowing them to decide whether to separate themselves from their child, or to have protected contact and "rooming in." Most parents opted for the latter. To be honest, we just did not know the right answer. Guidelines and recommendations can change time and again when we are dealing with a new disease and don't have complete information. But we did the best we could in a sea of uncertainty.

**On April 17, 2020**

- 2,196,109 cases of Covid-19 worldwide and 149,204 deaths.
- 672,303 cases of Covid-19 in the U.S. and 33,898 deaths.
- Hawaii closes all state beaches.
- A federal judge enters a temporary injunction against Genesis II Church of Health and Healing preventing sale of chlorine dioxide products, the equivalent of industrial bleach, as a Covid-19 treatment.

CHAPTER FOUR

# Innovation in the Time of Covid

*"What you are will show in what you do."*

**Thomas Edison**

Necessity is the mother of invention, and Covid-19 certainly created a lot of needs – the need for masks, the need for ventilators, and, as the number of patients grew, the seemingly never-ending need for additional negative pressure rooms. Into all of this stepped our problem solver: Steve Mosser, Holy Name's Executive Vice President of Operations.

A jack-of-all trades, Steve honed his natural problem-solving abilities during his time in the Merchant Marines. He and his crew would go to sea for months at a time, and Steve would fix any mechanical issues that arose with whatever he had on hand. He now uses this resourcefulness and outside-the-box thinking to run the hospital's day-to-day operations.

Steve oversees hundreds of employees. He runs our construction projects, ensures that the hospital complies with state and federal building regulations, negotiates leases and property sales, and even makes sure the boilers and the HVAC are always functioning properly. Steve guarantees that Holy Name is a safe and inviting space for our patients and our employees, and his job performance can directly impact patient care.

Such was the case during this unprecedented health crisis.

From the day we admitted our first Covid-19 patient, Steve's team worked as quickly as they could to convert rooms to negative pressure. But we were quickly running out of both rooms and time. Steve was extremely concerned that we were not going to be able to convert enough "regular" rooms to negative pressure rooms to keep up with the volume of Covid-19 patients being admitted. If his team couldn't keep up, care would be compromised, and we would be putting our staff at increased risk of being infected. He thought Covid-19 might overwhelm us. But he had an idea.

I brought Michele Acito, our acting Chief Nursing Officer (CNO) into the conversation, and Steve pitched us his idea: build an entire negative pressure ward that could house multiple beds within a single space. We were interested in the concept; negative pressure rooms, which contained just one bed each, were not an efficient use of space. But where could we put an entire negative pressure ward? According to Steve, in the storage space behind our operating room (OR). This space was the size of half a football field and packed with random pieces of hospital equipment: beds, operating microscopes, IV poles, office supplies, Christmas decorations, computers, and desks. Think of it as the hospital's equivalent of an attic.

Michele was particularly intrigued with Steve's idea. Typically, one critical care nurse covers one to two patients, but with a large, open space, and nurses working in teams, two critical care nurses could cover as many as six patients. This more efficient system would also allow Michele to pair her experienced critical care staff with those nurses who, while fully trained, had less hands-on experience.

I, on the other hand, had some reservations. The space was completely unfinished. It didn't even have real walls, just exposed studs lining the perimeter of the room. It was hardly a place I would want anyone in my own family to be treated – a standard I often apply when making decisions about the hospital. I expressed my concern, and Steve insisted that he could frame out the space to make it patient-friendly. I also admitted to myself that if the space were used for critically ill patients, the vast majority of them would not be alert enough to care about the amenities (not a thought I would have ever entertained if we were not in the middle of a crisis).

Mike, who was quarantining at home after his positive Covid-19 diagnosis, was not well enough to weigh in on this decision. His ability to run Holy Name during this challenging time lessened as his symptoms worsened. At first, we spoke to him daily and as often as needed. But over time, his health declined, and we called him for only the most crucial decisions. Eventually, he grew too fatigued to participate in any decision-making and he fully passed the baton to the rest of the management team.

As the CMO, the decision about converting the storage space was on me. The choice was a matter of weighing wants and needs. We may all have wanted a nicer space for our patients, but what we needed was more beds in negative pressure spaces. I did not see a better option. I gave Steve the go ahead to draw up a full plan.

He quickly turned his rough sketches into complete blueprints, laying out the floor plan, bed placement, and equipment for the new ward. Beyond his novel idea to convert the storage space into an entire unit for Covid-19 patients, Steve developed an innovative approach for the placement of the equipment needed to care for these patients. In a normal hospital room, the ventilators, IV pumps, and monitors are right next to the patient's bed, in close proximity to the patient. Steve wanted to build the new space so that most of the equipment – ventilators, IV pumps, and monitors – would be further from the patient, outside the immediate patient care area. This way, nurses could check and use this equipment without risking exposure to Covid-19.

We had started to implement a similar setup in the existing ICU by drilling through the walls of patients' rooms, but Steve felt that designing the new unit with this concept in mind would allow us to use the space more efficiently and more effectively. He asked for a day to consult with Greg Bozzo, an outside consultant who leads many of our construction projects, so that they could finalize a plan.

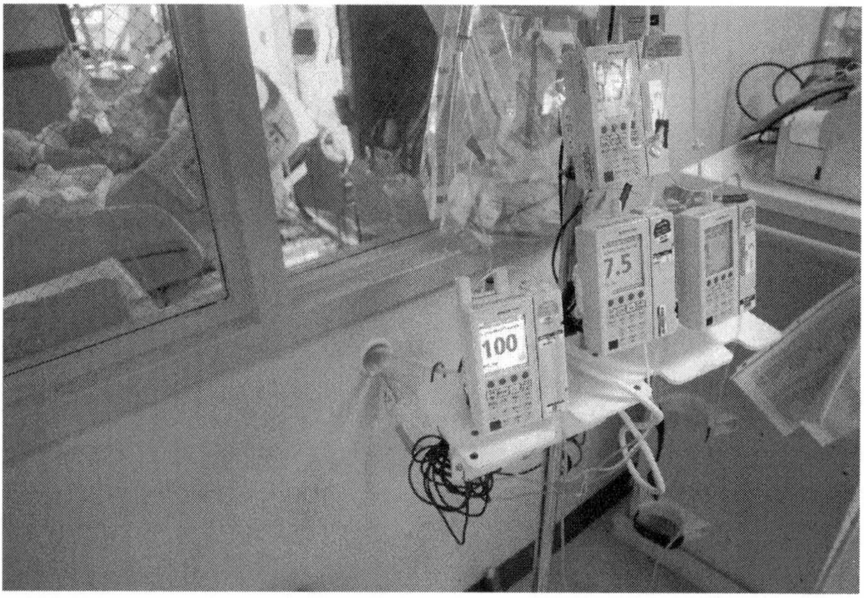


Holes were cut into the ICU walls so that IV units with pumps could be kept outside the patient's room, allowing for easy monitoring and adjusting by nurses and minimizing the need for PPE.

Steve envisioned one unit in the space with two separate wards, each with their own negative pressure systems and each of which could serve 15 to 20 patients. When we cleared out the room to simulate the placement of 20 beds (using tape on the floor), space was tight. Michele insisted that clinicians would not have adequate space to provide the necessary care with that many beds in the room, so we settled on 18 beds.

We began to call the unit "the Shell." Each ward in the unit would be a room within a room. The patients would be located in the inner room, with the head of each bed placed up against the wall like in a normal hospital room. Each bed would have a window above it, allowing nurses to observe their patients without entering the inner room. This entire inner ward would have negative pressure with no air (and no virus) escaping, except through the designated vents.

The inner room would be surrounded by corridors on all four sides, creating a larger room. It was in this outer room that the main equipment would be located, with just the tubing and monitoring lines from the equipment going into the central room through holes in the wall. This way, whenever a nurse needed to check an alarm or adjust an IV, the nurse would not need to enter the patient space. We knew that this would have a tremendous impact on our use of PPE and overall efficiency. In the other Covid-19 areas of the hospital, 80 percent of the time a nurse entered a patient's room, it was simply to check or adjust equipment. And each time, the nurse had to put on a fresh set of PPE. The small adjustment of moving the equipment outside the patient care area would drastically decrease our PPE use.

Additionally, Steve designed pass-through windows – cut outs in the walls that were covered by small plexiglass squares that could be lifted for access to the inner room. If a nurse in the room needed a piece of equipment, a medication, or a dressing, they could use a microphone to tell staff outside the Shell to pass it in – with no need to leave the room and no need to change PPE.

In a final stroke of genius, Steve decided to hang mirrors from the ceiling in front of each bed. His design placed patients' heads near the wall of the inner room to reduce the length of IV and ventilator tubing, but this meant that patients would face away from the windows – and that nurses would not be able to see their patients' faces. Using the mirrors, nurses could see their patients' reflections to assess their level of comfort or sedation. In a few cases, those mirrors were eventually replaced with cameras.

When we shared the plan to convert the storage space with Mike a few days after Steve proposed the idea, he was skeptical. At this point, he and his entire family had recovered, and Mike was back in charge, albeit via phone call (he still needed to quarantine). After hearing the plan, Mike made it clear that he wasn't on board with caring for patients in a "warehouse." To Mike, it simply wasn't in line with what people expected from Holy Name – even in the middle of a crisis. But Mike hadn't been at the hospital for almost two weeks. While he knew about the influx of patients on our doorstep, he hadn't yet seen the crisis in person. I knew firsthand what we were up against, and I was frustrated by his decision, even if I understood his concern.

We delayed the construction and spent the next three days looking for possible alternatives. On the fourth day, Mike was well enough to come back to the hospital. Two weeks normally might not seem like a lot of time to be away from the job, but in those two weeks, the world had turned upside down.

Upon his return, Mike was visibly struck by how the hospital had changed – the plastic sheeting where the doors used to be, the massive increase in Covid-19 patients, the staff fully attired in PPE. The outside world had come to a grinding halt as people sheltered at home, but the rush of activity within the hospital had grown at breakneck speed, and with it, an enormous weight had been placed on our entire staff as they tried to protect patients – and themselves – from this deadly virus.

We had described all of this to Mike, but mere words and numbers could not do it justice. After Mike saw the rest of the hospital, Steve gave Mike a tour of the storage space, explaining his vision. The look on Mike's face as he stood in the middle of the empty room said it all: we needed more beds, and we needed them now. Without hesitation, Mike agreed to proceed with the construction. Steve and his crew built out the new Covid-19 unit, capable of housing 36 patients, in just four days.

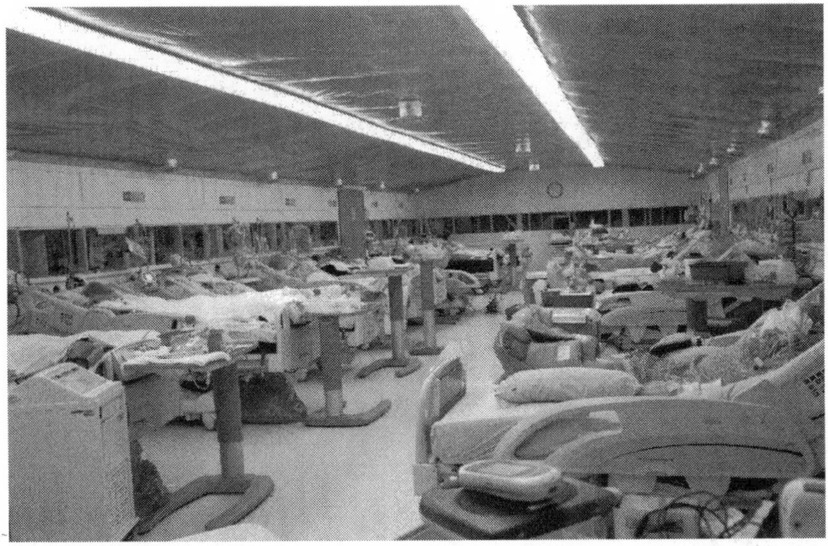

Holy Name's specially designed and built Covid-19 ward, known as "the Shell."

Portraits of masked staff lined the hallway leading to the Shell. A fantastic photographer who was part of our Holy Name team, Jeff Rhode, was on site every day. He provided video and pictures to television and magazines. Any in-hospital video of Holy Name that appeared on the local news – and on some of the national news – was likely shot by Jeff. Even much of the in-hospital footage from Bruce Springsteen's television fundraiser for the New Jersey Pandemic Relief Fund came from Jeff. He also took the photographs that appear in this book.

A month or two into the pandemic, Jeff shot a series of powerful black-and-white portraits – the ones leading to the Shell – of Holy Name staff in full PPE, with only their eyes visible. It is amazing how much of a person's humanity comes through in their eyes. When I gazed at those portraits, I saw a deep desire to help, along with a tinge of helplessness. Tears were not visible, but I could sense that they might not be far away.

We later moved these portraits to the entryway of our cafeteria to stand as tribute to our healthcare workers – or as some say, "the heroes without capes."

* * * * *

When the Shell received its first patient on April 3, just shy of one month after our first Covid-19 patient had arrived, we had 217 Covid-19-dedicated beds, 63 of which were for critically ill patients. The new wards were completed in the nick of time; we were just passing our 200-patient mark, and the new unit filled in a matter of days.

Two weeks later, as Steve made his daily rounds to see how the new wards were functioning, he walked into a scene of controlled chaos. Two teams of nurses, doctors, and technicians were diligently trying to save two patients who were in cardiac arrest – in adjacent beds. Team members rotated as they performed CPR. CPR is not the sanitized procedure that you see on television. It is an exhausting and, frankly, brutal process. The person giving CPR will put one hand over the other on the patient's chest and shove down with all their strength. With every push, the CPR administrator compresses the chest by about two inches, using enough force that some patients suffer a broken rib or two. Non-medical observers are often shocked by the seemingly violent procedure.

That day in the Covid-19 ward, each CPR team consisted of five people. Two anesthesiologists, one for each patient, squeezed cantaloupe-sized rubber bags, forcing oxygen into the patients' lungs and monitoring their airways. Two lead physicians stood on the other side of the beds, monitoring the patients' heart rhythms, overseeing the staff response to the code, and making second-by-second calls on what medicine, procedure, or test to do next. Nurses responded to the lead physicians, getting medications from the "code cart" and administering them through the patients' IV tubing. There was also a person assigned to each team documenting every action taken.

Steve had never seen CPR administered before. He paused in the doorway, a bit pale, turned to Michele, and said, "You were right. Good thing we didn't attempt to get more beds in here – there never would have been enough room."

One of those patients, despite the best efforts of the staff, did not make it through that day. The other did. Later that week, however, that patient died.

Even with the new Covid-19 ward, we still barely remained ahead of the need for negative pressure beds. We determined that the next ward should be built in Marian Hall, one of Holy Name's conference spaces. Marian Hall is an educational center that is used by physicians, nurses, other hospital staff, and the community. It was partially funded by a federal grant as part of a hospital expansion project after the September 11, 2001 attacks, and was designed for patient care in case of a serious emergency. This portion of the hospital has separate air flow, electric, and plumbing from the rest of the hospital, in case a situation ever arose where we needed to shelter in place. This past investment in preparation for a future disaster paid off for Holy Name and its patients during Covid-19.

As soon as the Shell was completed, Steve began construction of three additional wards in Marian Hall, each with a 20-patient capacity. Like the Shell, these wards had negative pressure, equipment outside the unit so that nurses could make adjustments without going into the space, pass throughs, and mirrors to easily see patients' faces. All three wards served both ICU and non-ICU patients as needed.

This newly renovated space is where we now treat all Covid-19 patients, as of November 2020. It's the perfect Covid-19 unit: isolated from the remainder of the hospital, cosmetically more appealing than the original Shell, and large enough to accommodate all our current Covid-19 patients. We hope that we will not need to return to the use of the Shell or other wards during the remainder of the pandemic, but as of publication, that seems optimistic.

Once the new units were up and running, our "bed crunch" dramatically improved. We had increased our Covid-19 capacity to more than 275 beds, from an original six. The flexibility that these additional wards gave us prevented what could have been a dire situation. Steve had shared a vision and got it done – improving the quality and efficiency of care for hundreds of patients.

Steve's innovations were not limited to construction of the Covid-19 wards. He also designed a personal negative pressure pod, which we called the ISO-pod.

ISO-pods were boxes made of plexiglass, with a top and sides but no bottom. They went from just above a patient's head to just above the knee. By the patient's head, each ISO-pod had a duct that sucked air from inside the container through a filter, creating a mini-negative pressure space that stopped air from escaping into the outside room. Each pod also had holes on the sides of the boxes big enough that nurses could reach through to provide necessary care to the patient.

We initially intended to isolate all suspected Covid-19 patients in single rooms, but that just wasn't feasible with the number of patients we admitted. ISO-pods allowed us to place two patients in a single negative pressure room while we were awaiting Covid-19 test results, which, at the time, took five to seven days to receive. The ability to put more than one patient in the same room without risking cross-infection thanks to the ISO-pods was a game changer.

I am not sure if Steve was a *Get Smart* fan, but if he was, the ISO-pods might have been inspired by the "cone of silence." But unlike the technology in the 1960s TV show, these pods actually worked.

As we do with much of our new technology, we tested the ISO-pods in our Simulation Center prior to using them with real patients. The Simulation Center allows us to replicate real-life situations by practicing on lifelike mannequins: they speak, their eyes react to light, they can be hooked up to IVs, and their skin can change color. We regularly use simulations to practice complex robotic surgery or patient-caregiver interactions. Simulations help build team cohesion and improve communication – which is an increasingly important skill, as the practice of medicine becomes more complex. For example, simulations have undoubtedly helped how our stroke and heart attack teams care for patients by improving response time in managing these medical conditions.

I've experienced the efficacy of the Simulation Center firsthand. One of our simulations aims to help staff and caregivers better understand how a patient with Alzheimer's experiences the world. Several years ago, I gave it a try to see if it could help me understand the struggles my father, who had dementia, experienced every day.

I was given glasses that blurred my sight, gloves to mimic loss of fine motor skills, and inserts in my shoes that generated the discomfort that certain Alzheimer's patients feel with neuropathy (foot pain). The main lights in the simulation room were lowered, strobe lights were turned on, and music was turned up loudly. I was then given 10 tasks to complete in 15 minutes – easy tasks, like sorting laundry, buttoning a shirt, or putting on a tie. Well, easy for most people. As I experienced a simulation of what Alzheimer's patients experience, I quickly became frustrated.

After experiencing this simulation, I found that I was much more patient and understanding when my dad had food on his clothes, or when his shirt buttons were in the wrong holes. The simulation had such a huge impact on me –

and my relationship with my father – that we decided that all staff who cared for dementia patients should experience it. Since we made this simulation part of the mandatory training for our caregivers, we have seen a significant improvement in the way Holy Name staff interact with this challenging group of patients.

Holy Name developed its Simulation Center after Mike and several other staff members toured Israel's top medical facilities in 2008. The trip included a stop at the Israel Center for Medical Simulation, founded by Dr. Amitai Ziv. The Center convinced the Holy Name team of the value of simulation-based training and soon after the trip, we opened our own Simulation Center at Holy Name.

We were lucky that Angelica Berrie, President of the Russell Berrie Foundation and widow of Russell Berrie, joined the Holy Name staff in Israel. Russell Berrie was a big name in toys for decades, and became one of the most innovative philanthropists of his time. When a child is in the hospital, the perfect gift to cheer them up is a teddy bear; when you are a major developer and seller of specialty bears, the perfect gift for a hospital is a simulation center. Angelica Berrie and the Foundation's support goes beyond the Simulation Center. When we decided to close the hospital's kitchen to minimize food service workers interactions with other staff, they generously provided pre-packaged meals for our entire staff, and continued to do this throughout the first wave of the pandemic.

When Steve built the first ISO-pod, I was skeptical that it would work in real life, so I was eager to test it in the Simulation Center. When I walked in, a large group of people were gathered around a mannequin inside an ISO-pod. I had planned to watch quietly, but my skepticism got the better of me when I saw the holes in the sides of the ISO-pods. "Steve," I blurted out, "this isn't airtight. It's not even close."

"Don't worry," Steve said. "The pod doesn't have to be airtight, it just has to draw a steady flow of air into the pod and out through the duct."

I raised my eyebrows, still unconvinced, and Steve laughed. "You're a doctor, not an engineer, dammit!" He knew a Star Trek reference would win me over. "Just stay in your lane."

With that, he pulled out a bottle and sprayed a fine white powder into one of the holes on the side of the pod.

As intended, the powder was quickly pulled out of the pod, then into the duct and out of the room through a filter – simulating the path of an aerosolized virus emitted from a patient. The same thing happened when he sprayed the powder into the larger opening over the mannequin's legs. This was much further from the duct, but Steve knew that the negative pressure would easily do the job. He looked pleased; he had done it again. I reminded myself to trust my team and, as Steve so eloquently put it, to "stay in my lane."

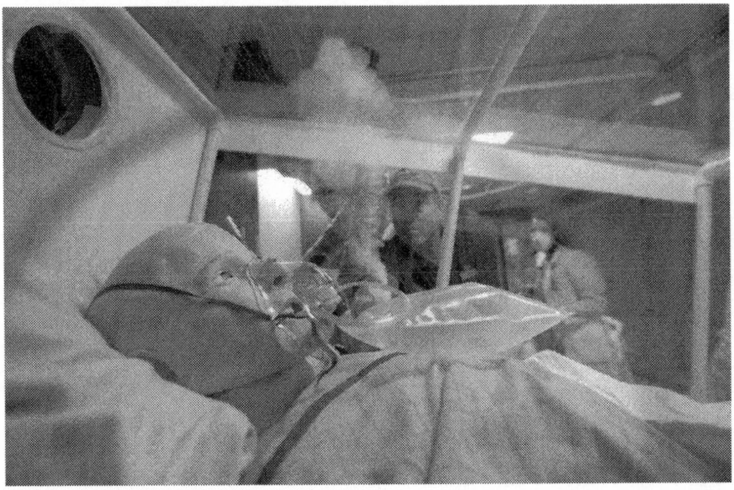

Steve testing an ISO-pod in the Holy Name Simulation Center.

After testing the ISO-pods on mannequins, we successfully tested them on hospital volunteers before going into full production. Steve immediately sent his team out across multiple states to gather the materials he needed – plexiglass,

HVAC ducts, fans, and other components. Steve and his dedicated staff then started building, making more than 200 ISO-pods in just a few days.

The only flaw in the ISO-pods' design was that they were heavy, and nurses struggled to move them to allow patients to exercise or use the bathroom. So, we developed a new job: pod movers. A group of physical therapists who were not seeing patients during Covid-19 agreed to move the pods when needed. As an added benefit, these therapists developed special exercises for those in ISO-pods as they interacted with those patients.

The ISO-pods were a resounding success. Patients tolerated them well, staff and patients both felt better protected when they were used, and they allowed us to place multiple patients in one room. Most importantly, I am convinced that they kept staff from getting infected. Steve's two innovations – "the Shell" concept and the ISO-pods – saved lives. We tried to publicize the ISO-pods' success and share their construction plans, hoping that other hospitals would adopt this essential technology. We made YouTube videos. We discussed it in our daily calls with other area hospitals. I tried to plug it on CNN. Despite our best efforts, other hospitals did not follow our lead. These may have been outside-the-box ideas, but other hospitals were not willing to try something new and unproven, even if it meant saving lives.

* * * * *

Throughout this whole terrible ordeal, we raced against time – could we add beds fast enough to meet the number of patients being admitted? Even with the addition of the ISO-pods, it seemed that as soon as new beds were ready, patients arrived to fill them. At our peak, on April 13, we had 251 Covid-19 patients, with 45 on ventilators. We had the capacity for 276 Covid-19 patients – a safety net of 25 beds, which we thankfully never had to use. In the end, with the help of engineers, carpenters, and trained staff, we stayed at least one hour ahead

– and sometimes only an hour.

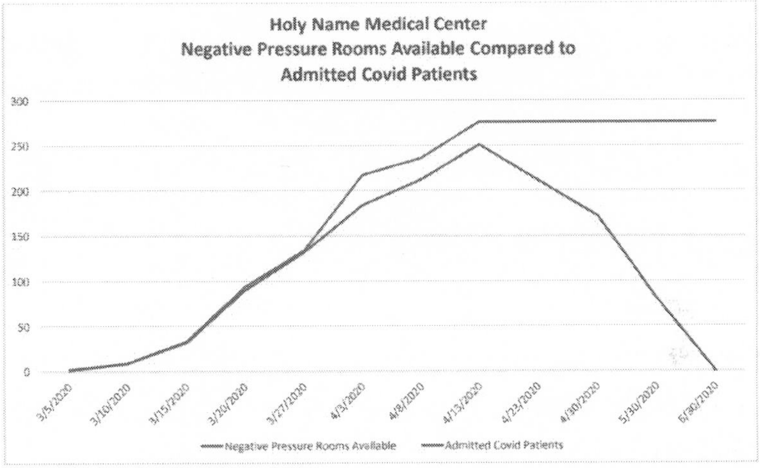

CHAPTER FIVE

# What We Know and What We Don't Know

*"I am the wisest man alive, for I know one thing,*
*and that is that I know nothing."*

**Plato**
The Republic
375 BC

A few days prior to the CNN interview, Michele noticed that Mike seemed "off." She brought this to my attention and she and I, with another nursing leader, Cedar Wang, approached him.

"Mike, we don't want to overstep, but you don't seem yourself. Are you feeling okay?"

Mike shrugged. "I'm a little tired, but aren't we all?" He didn't have any known Covid-19 symptoms: no coughing, no trouble breathing, no sore throat. We weren't too worried, but the four of us made a pact that day. We would report any Covid-19 symptoms to each other immediately.

We knew that if any or all of us got sick, the hospital might not have the leadership it needed to get through this crisis. We were worried about each other's health, but just as much, we were worried about the hospital.

We still do not and never will know if Mike's fatigue was an initial symptom of Covid-19. Nor do we know how or where Mike got infected, or whether he infected his wife, or his wife infected him. That is one of the many challenges of this disease. Patients can present with very mild symptoms or, as we later learned, with no symptoms at all, making it very difficult to track the spread of the disease.

I did not get Covid-19 (at least not to my knowledge). Not from the days I spent with Mike, nor from the days I spent at the hospital with as many as 251 Covid-19 patients. Nor when I worked alongside doctors and nurses who got infected. One of the mysteries of Covid-19, at least for now, is why some people get it and others in the same situation do not.

Entire families have been infected, one family member after another. For example, the Fuscos, a family in New Jersey, had seven infections. Grace Fusco, mother of 11 and grandmother of 27, died on a ventilator unaware that her two oldest children had already died of the disease. In total, four Fusco family members died within one week.

Yet there were other cases where only one member of a family became infected, despite having been in close proximity to other members of the household day in and day out. Additionally, some people who cared for a loved one with Covid-19, even cradling them in their arms, never contracted the disease.

We do know that both length and intensity of exposure can impact transmission. When someone with Covid-19 who is highly contagious sneezes on you, this considerably raises the risk that you will get infected – but you still might not get it. Being in a confined room with someone ill with Covid-19 also increases your risk. In May, the *New York Times* profiled a church choir that continued to rehearse at the start of the pandemic, packed tightly together and singing gustily for two and a half hours. One of the members was symptomatic and, in hindsight, clearly contagious. That person later tested positive for Covid-19, as did 52 other choir members, a full 85 percent of those in attendance that evening. Two died. However, the remaining eight members who attended that rehearsal did not become ill.

It is possible that some people have not contracted Covid-19 (and never will) because they have "inherited immunity" – they were born with a trait that prevents Covid-19 infection. Others may have "acquired immunity"– immunity developed after birth. Those who survive Covid-19 develop acquired immunity to the disease, but it is still unclear how long this immunity lasts. Acquired immunity to Covid-19 may also occur from previous non-Covid-19 infections or from other factors, but we don't yet know why or how.

I have often wondered how I have escaped this virus so far. Have I developed immunity through years of patient exposure to similar viruses? Do I have some genetic inherent immunity? Could the flu shot I have taken for the past 30 years have built up a Covid-19 immunity? Am I extra careful about washing my hands and not touching my face? Or have I just been lucky? I don't know. It is even possible, though not likely, that I am one of the many folks who had an asymptomatic or very mild Covid-19 infection, but by the time I was tested for antibodies, they had dissipated.

The same questions apply to my hospital colleagues who have also escaped infection thus far. By the end of the first wave of Covid-19, Holy Name had 325 known staff members who had contracted Covid-19. We believe that the vast majority were infected in the community – through contact with friends, family, or strangers encountered outside of work – because of the precautions we have taken at Holy Name, but there is no way to be sure. We always return to the same point: we still do not know why some people get infected and others do not.

What we do know is that a person's current state of health can greatly impact the severity of the disease. A healthy 42-year-old who gets infected will probably feel lousy for a few weeks, akin to having a bad flu. A 62-year-old with severe emphysema, on the other hand, will likely (but not necessarily) require hospitalization, and might die. However, there have been cases of young, healthy people getting very sick and even dying – an extremely troubling occurrence that we often cannot explain. Other times, patients think they have no underlying health issues, but discover that they have diabetes or another undiagnosed chronic illness when they contract Covid-19.

Having an underlying chronic condition such as diabetes or cancer or being on certain medications that suppress the immune system are clear risk factors that can contribute to a more severe case of Covid-19. Weight seems to matter as well. Early in this pandemic when we saw healthy people who were just 15 to 20 pounds overweight admitted to the hospital, already in great distress, we knew that this was not a typical "flu-like illness." These patients not only became more gravely ill than those who were not overweight, but had a higher mortality rate as well.

I have two theories as to why central obesity (sometimes described as "a tire around the middle") affects a patient's Covid-19 trajectory. Either it is tied to, or correlated with, a hyper-immune response (when the immune system becomes so active that it causes damage to parts of the body, like in auto-immune diseases such as rheumatoid arthritis or lupus). Or the extra weight inhibits lung capacity (overweight patients may not be able to breathe sufficiently deeply, which decreases the ability to get oxygen into the lungs). Or it could be both. This could also be why we see more men than women become critically ill with Covid-19, since men are more prone to central obesity. Without addressing the relationship between health and weight in general, in terms of Covid-19, it makes sense to be aware of your weight to decrease your risk of becoming severely ill.

How do all of these factors – inherent immunity, acquired immunity, and underlying health conditions – come together when evaluating the likelihood and severity of Covid-19 infections? We still don't know, but we have seen the disease impact certain communities more than others. For example, it has hit specifically the Black and Latinx communities harder than the general population. Perhaps Black and Latinx people are more genetically susceptible to Covid-19, but the higher infection and mortality rate is more likely caused by these communities' lack of access to healthcare, the fact that people of color are more likely to live in urban areas where it is harder to socially distance, and that a high percentage of our frontline workers are Black and Latinx. It also might be related to a higher prevalence of underlying conditions in these communities, which is primarily driven by a systemic lack of access to healthcare.

* * * * *

Throughout the pandemic, I found myself educating and advising staff, colleagues, and local community members such as our congressman, the local mayor, and religious leaders. I shared information with the general public as well, through radio and television interviews. These conversations often took me on interesting side journeys and sometimes along the way, while educating others, I learned a few things myself.

For the most part, these appearances were on news networks like CNN, CBS Radio, and many local networks. But one day, the hospital received a call from *Ed Randall's Talking Baseball*, a long-running chat radio program on WFAN in New York that focuses on the impact of baseball on our lives and culture, rather than current events in the game itself.

When our publicist Jessica asked if I wanted to be a guest on *Talking Baseball*, I quickly said yes. I've always enjoyed listening to the show. She added just as quickly that I would not be on to talk about baseball: the episode would be strictly Covid-19-related, and Ed's regular audience could call in and ask questions about the virus.

I was a little disappointed. I've been a baseball fan my whole life. I grew up watching professional games with my father, and I played Little League. When I was nine, I had a particularly great coach. He loved the game, he was extremely competitive, and his team always won. As it turned out, he would later become my father-in-law. I probably ran into Eileen that season – she would run around the park while her father and brothers were on the baseball field – but neither of us remember the other from that time. However, eight years later when she told her parents that we were going on our first date, her father definitely remembered me: "Nice kid, lousy baseball player." Still, I loved the game.

The day I appeared on *Talking Baseball*, Ed dove right in. "There has never been anything like this in our country in the past 100 years," he started. "It's been a week and a half since the World Health Organization (WHO) declared coronavirus a global pandemic." After he detailed the exponentially rising case count in New York City – it had more than quadrupled in a matter of days, and New York City had about 30 percent of the country's cases at that time – he introduced me as the episode's "leadoff hitter." I have to admit, my stomach fluttered.

After Ed and I spent a few minutes discussing Covid-19 and how Holy Name was handling it, he opened up the phone line for questions from listeners. At first, I fielded what were becoming standard Covid-19 questions. "How can I avoid getting it?" "Can I visit my relatives?" "Can I travel?" "What's going on at the hospital?"

And then we got an unusual call. "My daughter says she has 'Covid toes.' Is that a thing?" My first instinct was to say that was crazy, but I refrained – which was fortunate. Instead, I told the caller that I wasn't familiar with the condition but would do some research.

At the time, good medical information on Covid-19 was scarce, even in the medical journals. When I finished my appearance on *Talking Baseball*, I

Googled "Covid toes" to see what would come up. And there they were, pictures of very red, inflamed toes. Unlike gout, which affects the big toe, Covid toes appeared to mainly affect the little digits. I was genuinely surprised, and really glad that I had not told the caller that Covid toes were ridiculous.

When I got to the hospital later that day, I asked the nurses if they had seen Covid toes. While they had not seen the condition at our hospital, Michele said her 22-year-old niece had had a mild case of Covid-19 and did in fact have Covid toes. I asked if I could see them. Two hours later, Michele's niece, who had completely recovered except for her feet, arrived at the hospital lobby, where she took off her shoes and showed me her toes. They looked just like the pictures on Google. Although they were red and inflamed, they were not causing her any discomfort, and they later gradually returned to normal without any intervention.

My guess is that Covid toes are related to a post-infectious inflammatory response. It seems to occur in patients mostly after the acute infection subsides and may be related to micro-clotting, clotting that blocks the smallest veins or arteries leading to or from the skin of the small digits. This micro-clotting can lead to swelling and, in some rare cases, the need to remove the toe or toes.

By the way, my appearance on *Talking Baseball* garnered more compliments than any other appearance or interview I have done – I heard from family, friends, coworkers, and even a nun – one of the St. Joseph's Sisters of Peace, and an avid baseball fan.

Our introduction to Covid toes typified the way much of the information about the disease flowed early on – communication was very informal, and information was often garnered firsthand. One day out of the blue, I received a call from an NYU hematologist/oncologist, Dr. Michael Grossbard. He had seen a large number of Covid-19 patients who had developed complications related to clotting, so he had decided to call other hospitals in the New York area to tell them to be on the lookout. He didn't have to do this – it wasn't going to help his patients. But he wanted to get the word out to other healthcare providers as soon as possible.

We would have noticed the clotting issue eventually or been told through formal channels, but this early call put it on our radar sooner. Later that day, during a call I had with the heads of medicine at several Northern New Jersey hospitals, I passed along the concern. Since we had so little scientifically-tested knowledge of the disease, we used this type of anecdotal, person-to-person or hospital-to-hospital communication to learn from each other and to improve the quality of care for our patients.

Even in normal circumstances, hospitalized patients are prone to abnormal clotting, primarily related to two factors: 1) the body's increased production of certain clotting proteins during an acute illness, and 2) decreased mobility that occurs in most hospitalized patients. With Covid-19, the amount of clotting that we noticed was even higher than would have been expected. Autopsies of our Covid-19 patients confirmed our anecdotal evidence. Typically, we look for and detect clotting in the lungs with a CT scan, but this test cannot be performed in a patient's room, and it is challenging to move infectious patients who are on ventilators. Instead, we tested all critically ill patients with bedside ultrasounds to look for clots in the legs.

As the prevalence of clotting became more apparent, we weighed the risk of our patients developing clots against the risk of testing and treating them using preventative measures. Ultimately, we decided that the risk of clotting outweighed the risk of testing and treatment. Holy Name, like most hospitals, put almost all Covid-19 inpatients on blood thinners, at doses adjusted for the patient's level of illness. Administering blood thinner medications was the right decision. It saved lives. But it wasn't without risk. Blood thinners put patients at increased risk for bleeding, and we did have some Covid-19 patients who had bleeding in the gastrointestinal tract or the brain. As much as patients and their families look to medical professionals for black and white answers, medicine is complicated and often imprecise. Physicians and nurses must weigh the risks and benefits of every decision, many of which are not clear cut, especially with critically ill patients – and especially with a new disease when we have no choice but to learn on the job.

While we did our best with what we knew at the time, in hindsight, we sometimes made the wrong decision. For example, early on, based on information we had received from China and Europe, most hospitals and physicians decided to put patients on ventilators relatively early in the course of their infection. The goal was to get a patient on the ventilator in a controlled way, rather than wait until a patient was in crisis and needed to be put on the ventilator in a rush to save their life. Waiting to put a patient on a ventilator until the last possible moment increases the risks all around: a patient may be deprived of oxygen for too long, and the staff may have inadequate time to put on PPE.

But successfully getting patients off ventilators proved so difficult that, over time, medical consensus changed, and we now try to keep patients off ventilators as long as possible. A significant number of patients who ended up on ventilators did not survive, and our experience suggests that using all possible methods to avoid putting patients on ventilators has decreased the overall mortality rate. It did increase the mortality rate for people who went on ventilators, because those who were on ventilators were the sickest, and therefore the most likely to die. The decision to put a Covid-19 patient on a ventilator was a fine line to walk – and we got better at knowing when, and when not, to put someone on a ventilator as the crisis progressed.

Sometimes, very sick patients on ventilators can make an abrupt recovery, and we don't always know why. One day, a patient who had been on a ventilator for more than two weeks began to show slight signs of improvement, and then rather suddenly woke up. He was removed from the ventilator and, surprisingly, was immediately able to speak very clearly. The first thing he said was, "I need my phone so I can call my boss." He clearly had no idea how much time had passed.

"Your boss knows where you are. Call your wife," the nurse said, as she handed him a phone.

After a short, emotional call to his wife, he slowly looked around the room at the 17 other ventilated patients and asked the nurse, "Are those people going to be okay?"

This was a difficult question to answer then, and it remains a difficult question today. Even when a Covid-19 patient recovers from the disease, its long-term impact remains unknown. Caregivers have begun to use a new term for patients with chronic complications from Covid-19: "long haulers." Certainly, patients who require long-term ventilator support, as is the case for many critically ill Covid-19 patients, are at risk for neurological compromise, skin breakdown, and secondary pneumonias. While it is too soon to know if Covid-19 can cause long-term complications even for those who were not critically ill, I expect that it can. We have seen Covid-19 cause lung scarring and heart damage, which lead to shortness of breath and curtail the ability to exercise. We don't know whether full respiratory recovery will ever occur for some of these patients, and we will need to continue to study long haulers to provide them the most effective care possible.

Covid-19 is in many ways a masquerader. Based on our limited early understanding of the virus, we were expecting patients to present primarily with respiratory symptoms like nasal congestion, cough, or shortness of breath. But early on, one patient had us scratching our heads. He came in with extreme belly pain and diarrhea – but no respiratory issues at all. His Covid-19 test results came back positive. Several others with the same symptoms and the same test results followed in the next few weeks.

Covid-19 can also cause some people to temporarily lose the ability to taste and smell. This is likely related to the virus's impact on nerves in the nasal passageways. One teenager remarked that, for weeks, his food tasted like cardboard. As with Covid toes, my reaction to this symptom was initial skepticism. How many more things was this virus going to do – even if only in a few patients? And equally confusingly, why did some patients show no symptoms at all?

We also do not yet know the impact of Covid-19 on the brain. Relatives of some who have recovered say that their family members are not as sharp as they were before the infection took hold. Some call this "Covid brain fog." When the brain is hurt by a critical illness, it takes time to heal and bounce back, like an injured muscle. In some people, especially the young and healthy, this happens quickly. In older patients, it takes longer. In some already experiencing mental decline, it may mean that they never fully return to their previous cognitive level. Any significant hospital stay can negatively impact cognitive levels in patients with dementia, but it seems to be worse in Covid-19 patients. I am not sure if Covid brain fog is a result of the virus itself, micro-clotting in the brain caused by the virus, or something else entirely.

Perhaps Covid brain fog is caused by the treatment of the disease rather than the disease itself. Being on a ventilator is not a pleasant experience. Many patients on ventilators are in obvious physical discomfort, with a tube lodged in their throat and oxygen forced into their lungs. Most require sedation and paralyzation with a form of curare, the same substance traditionally used in poisoned darts. Long-term sedation and paralyzation increase the risk of complications, including potential issues with cognition.

* * * * *

While patients who survive Covid-19 have some degree of immunity, we have seen patients return to the hospital with recurrent symptoms, weeks to months after their initial infection. We don't know if they have been reinfected, or if they are returning with symptoms related to the initial infection, or even if these are symptoms completely unrelated to Covid-19. We have learned that even after a patient has recovered from an acute infection, they can retain non-infectious remnants of Covid-19 RNA in their naso-pharynx, the upper part of the throat behind the nose. The most reliable testing for Covid-19 does not differentiate viable infectious RNA from this remnant non-infectious RNA. While a more detailed genetic analysis of the Covid-19 virus can make this differentiation, this test is not routinely available in hospitals. The bottom line is that routine testing does not tell us whether patients have a new infection or have persistent symptoms related to a previous infection.

Our bodies are amazing. They respond quickly and, usually, very effectively to things that they are not familiar with, be it a virus, bacteria, or allergen, such as pollen. One of our major response mechanisms is to generate antibodies that attack these intruders. If the body's initial response is successful, the next time the same intruder presents itself, the body reacts more quickly and more effectively.

This is why vaccines work. We create and introduce to the body a version of an intruder that is relatively harmless, but that triggers the production of antibodies. This process teaches the body how to fight the real intruder at a later point if necessary. This same response is what causes acquired immunity.

For some diseases, like measles, immunity lasts a lifetime for most patients. For other diseases, it can last for just a year or even less. And the duration of the immunity can vary from person to person.

So, what about Covid-19? To learn more about the possible duration of immunity, we tested staff who had suffered acute infections for antibody levels immediately after their recovery, then retested them over time to follow their antibody levels.

Unfortunately, the results of our testing were not encouraging. One nurse had high levels of antibodies for a few weeks after her recovery, but when she was retested six weeks later, the antibodies were completely gone. Other staff members did not have as dramatic a drop in their levels, but we consistently saw a decrease in antibody levels over time.

Whether resistance to reinfection by Covid-19 will last a few months or for years will play a major role in the development of a vaccine that can allow us to truly return to our normal lives. My guess, based on these antibody test results, is that a Covid-19 infection does not generate long-term immunity. We will likely need an annual vaccine, similar to the flu shot, rather than a lifetime vaccine, like the one for chickenpox.

Even after reviewing all these unknowns – Covid toes, blood clotting, loss of taste and smell, impaired brain function, and immunity – there is still one more long-term effect that bears mentioning: post-traumatic stress disorder (PTSD). We don’t know how many patients will suffer Covid-19-related PTSD or how severe their symptoms will be, but being on a ventilator in an ICU or facing death away from family is incredibly stressful and traumatic. Physicians who care for patients who have recovered from Covid-19 must be aware that their patients are at increased risk of PTSD, and must be prepared to treat it. Some family members of infected patients will also suffer from PTSD as a result of Covid-19. And, of course, this pandemic will have a huge psychological impact on our healthcare providers. Hospitals and other medical employers must be ready to provide the support their staff needs when working in a psychologically distressing environment – something I had experienced before when working on an AIDS ward in the late 1980s and early 1990s.

**On June 5, 2020**

- 6.6 million cases worldwide.
- WHO urges all governments to encourage their citizens to wear masks.
- The University of Pennsylvania makes the SAT/ACT optional for applicants due to concerns about the spread of Covid-19 at standardized testing sites.

CHAPTER SIX

# Lessons from the AIDS Pandemic

*"This is tangible to the mainstream in a way that AIDS wasn't.
We had preachers on television telling us every day that
this was God's punishment to us.
Now, there is none of that. This new health crisis applies to everyone."*

**Mark S. King**
HIV/AIDS Activist
March 23, 2020

I attended medical school at George Washington University in Washington, D.C. At that time, the incidence of HIV/AIDS in D.C. was still quite small, so I had minimal exposure to the disease during my medical school training.

In 1985, my first year of medical school, there were 15,527 known cases of HIV/AIDS in the U.S. Four years later when I started my residency in New York City, there were over 100,000 cases in the U.S. New York City had roughly 20 percent of them. I found myself thrust into the middle of a brutal health crisis – the HIV/AIDS pandemic.

Medical school graduates are credentialed doctors, but after graduating, they must first serve a year as an intern at a hospital under the supervision of more senior physicians. Then, depending on what specialty they choose, they spend an additional two to five years as a resident.

An intern is not licensed as a physician, but a resident has all the rights and privileges of being a doctor. Residents rotate through different hospital wards, work alongside experienced doctors, and grapple with real problems.

Medical school teaches you theory, but residency teaches you how to put that theory into practice.

Residents are responsible for the care of a specific group of assigned patients. During my years as a primary care/internal medicine resident from 1989 to 1992, I was assigned to New York Hospital's AIDS ward approximately 30 percent of the time. During those weeks, two other residents and I oversaw 8 to 12 patients each. Ninety percent of the patients were gay men, though there was an occasional woman or straight man who had contracted HIV/AIDS from drug use, a blood transfusion, or heterosexual sex.

During the second and third year of my residency, every day I gathered for a morning report with 12 fellow residents and a Senior Attending Physician. The morning report was a high-pressure meeting in which we were grilled on patients we had admitted overnight and on the decisions we had made regarding their care. While stressful, the morning report certainly motivated us to learn as much as possible about our patients' illnesses. Even after a long shift, residents often hit the Cornell library to review their case documents and read about their patients' illnesses in preparation for our morning report. No one wanted to be tripped up by some obscure or minor fact.

Lining one wall of the meeting room were photographs of all the previous Chief Residents, staring down as if compelling the current residents to carry on the long tradition of providing the highest quality of care. At New York Hospital, the Chief Resident was a physician who had completed both their residency and one to two years of fellowship training in a subspecialty before being appointed Chief Resident by the Chief of Medicine and the Residency Committee. The Chief Resident's primary responsibility was to ensure that the residents had an exceptional educational experience. Only the best of the best were appointed Chief Resident at New York Hospital – it was a very prestigious position.

Most of the pictures on the wall belonged to nameless faces who, while they had probably gone on to distinguished careers in medicine, were unknown to the current residents. But there was one face we all knew: Dr. Anthony Fauci, one of our own who was a national leader in the fight against HIV/AIDS as the Director of the National Institute of Allergy and Infectious Diseases. We spoke of him and the work he was doing with a sort of whispered reverence. It made us all proud to think that he had spent his time as a resident sitting in this room and walking the same halls we did.

When Dr. Fauci again came into the public eye during the Covid-19 pandemic, I was publicly relieved, and again, quietly proud. I have never met Dr. Fauci, but for decades now, I have known of his reputation as a brilliant, tireless physician who always put the patient first. I had confidence that if he was allowed to lead, the U.S. would make the right decisions and get through this pandemic with as little loss of life as possible.

In the beginning of the HIV/AIDS pandemic (as with the Covid-19 pandemic), we did not have a definitive treatment. Now, treatment for AIDS is fairly standard, but we are still trying to determine the best treatment for Covid-19. On the other hand, while a vaccine for Covid-19 seems likely, we still do not have one for HIV/AIDS (though not for lack of trying).

Despite these differences, the diseases have noteworthy similarities. Both diseases can be prevented by making changes in our day-to-day behavior, like wearing condoms (to prevent HIV/AIDS) and washing your hands (to prevent Covid-19). For the most part, neither disease has had a particularly strong impact on the very young. One very dangerous similarity is that HIV, like Covid-19, can be spread when someone does not have any symptoms, allowing it to stealthily take root in a community. With both diseases, this contributed to a delayed response by public health officials.

We couldn't cure HIV/AIDS when I encountered it during residency – we still can't – but we got very good at treating complications that often developed, primarily opportunistic infections (diseases that take advantage of a weakened immune system) such as pneumocystis pneumonia and toxoplasmosis. Our patients would often get well enough to go home, but every time we discharged a patient, we knew they would be back in a few months with another complication. Some patients left the ward as many as three or four times before they left for good.

* * * * *

Over time, many of the residents, myself included, became friendly with our HIV/AIDS patients and their partners (some of whom would later enter the ward themselves). I became close with one patient in particular, Thomas. He was in his late 20s, about my age, and had an endless barrage of medical questions – much more than the average patient. He explained that his mother had always wanted him to be a doctor, but that he had gone into the arts instead. I related – I became a doctor largely because of my own mother's wishes, even though I had loved theater and performing when I was younger. Thomas had always thought he could go back to school if his first career didn't work out, but now he knew he would never have that chance.

As Thomas neared the end of his life, he was no longer able to make his own decisions about his care. Even today, most patients do not have a healthcare proxy. HIV/AIDS patients were even less likely to have one, because they had not expected to face end-of-life medical decisions at such a young age. Since most HIV/AIDS patients could not legally marry their partners, decision making responsibility transferred to the next of kin, usually a parent. In Thomas's case, this was his father.

Thomas's parents did not accept his sexual orientation and openly blamed Thomas's significant other, Stan, for infecting and endangering their son. When Thomas became incapable of making decisions regarding his own care, it didn't take long for Thomas's father to exert his new authority by banning Stan from the room during Thomas's slow drift to death. What I witnessed was an ugly, painful confrontation resulting in Stan being physically removed from the hospital room. There was no way the medical staff could legally intervene. It was cruel and unbearably sad – and it was far too common a scene during the years that I took care of patients on the ward.

Too many HIV/AIDS patients died separated from those they loved, and too many of their loved ones were robbed of the opportunity to say goodbye. As I watched our Covid-19 patients succumb to the virus without their loved ones by their side, images from the AIDS ward 30 years earlier flashed through my mind. This was a different disease, a different reason for separating patients from their families. But I was haunted by the similarities: patients sick, scared, and alone.

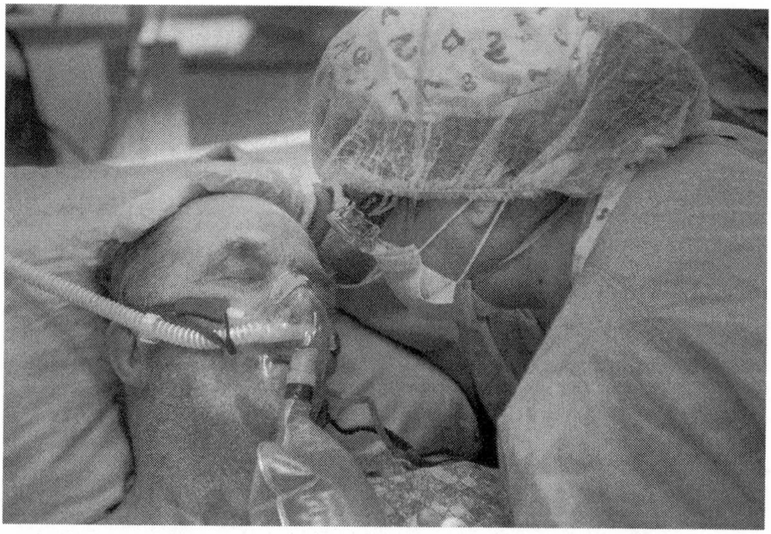

One of the cruelest aspects of Covid-19: patients dying without their families by their side. A strain on both families and healthcare workers.

In 1985, a *Los Angeles Times* poll found that a majority of Americans were in favor of quarantining people with HIV/AIDS. Like HIV/AIDS, Covid-19 led to stigmatization of and prejudice against groups thought to be associated with the disease. It is difficult to compare the society-wide discrimination against gay men and others with HIV/AIDS to discrimination faced by other groups. But we must acknowledge that Asian Americans have faced increased, unfounded, racial harassment due to the Covid-19 pandemic.

On an individual basis, many Covid-19 patients have faced stigmatization borne out of fear of becoming infected. In several cases, we had patients who were ready to be discharged from the hospital and return home – to a home shared with relatives. Their families wanted them to stay in the hospital. We explained to family members that their loved ones were likely not infectious ("likely," because in healthcare there are very few absolutes) and that they could not remain in the hospital. It was just not feasible to use the hospital as a quarantine facility. There were too many acute patients who needed care, and for most patients, home quarantine was a reasonable and safe option. Eventually, we convinced the reluctant families to bring their loved ones home. But this aggressive fighting of the patient's wishes to return home often caused hard feelings that I suspect impacted emotional, and possibly physical, recovery for the patient.

As with Covid-19, working on the AIDS ward could be overwhelming. Young people were dying. At that time, HIV/AIDS had a 100 percent mortality rate. I remember looking out over the AIDS ward, thinking, "All of these people are going to die." Many of us on the staff suffered some degree of PTSD.

It is likely that some healthcare workers who live through this pandemic and who have cared for Covid-19 patients will also suffer from PTSD. As previously mentioned, patients who survive Covid-19 are at risk as well.

PTSD affects people in different ways, but typically it disrupts sleep and causes severe anxiety or depression. It can be a devastating disease to live with.

In the late '80s and early '90s, it felt like doctors and nurses toiled alone on the front lines fighting HIV/AIDS and caring for patients. It wasn't until nearly five years after the first known case in the United States that President Ronald Reagan even mentioned AIDS in a public forum. But with Covid-19, my staff never felt alone. To the contrary, we felt truly appreciated. At the hospital, front line workers received unexpected food deliveries for the night shift, donations of Girl Scout cookies, and drawings from children. One afternoon, a parade of fire engines and police cars circled the hospital, sirens and horns blaring, lights flashing, and arms extended from windows holding handmade signs of support.

Throughout the entire community, the displays of gratitude – signs on lawns and in store windows – did not go unnoticed. They were truly a welcomed source of motivation as I drove to work each morning, and a welcomed source of comfort on the way home.

Towards the end of March, I arrived home one Friday evening shortly before 7 p.m., and after a quick shower, sat down on the couch, my new place of residence as Eileen and I attempted to social distance from one another. I opened up my laptop to check in on the hospital. Every night, I received an onslaught of emails and phone calls to return. Frequently, an additional crisis had developed during my short drive home.

I turned on the news, while Eileen opened one of the living room windows wide and told me she was going up to the roof for a few minutes. I didn't think much of this; our apartment is often warm, even in the cooler months, and Eileen loves to watch the sun set from the roof.

A few minutes later, I heard a sound drifting in through the window. In

New York City, it's not unusual to hear traffic from the streets, or other loud noises. But this was different. The volume increased slowly and steadily, and as I raised my head toward the opened window, I could clearly hear people clapping, hooting, and banging pots. When I looked out the window, I could see Eileen up on the roof with her own metal cup, clanging away. She was by herself, but I saw others hanging out their windows, standing on fire escapes and cheering from their own rooftops. People in the streets below stopped in their tracks and applauded.

After about 10 minutes, Eileen returned to the apartment and asked, "Did you hear that? That was for *you*." She was actually a little choked up. I was, too.

Earlier in the month, Europeans in cities hit hard by Covid-19 had begun to show their appreciation for healthcare workers by applauding every evening. Now, New Yorkers were joining the movement to say "thank you."

I wasn't usually home early enough to hear the cheering in New York City, but it happened in Teaneck, too. Every night, for months, the entire community would come together to remind its healthcare workers that their work was not going unnoticed.

As we head into the winter months, it's quiet at 7 p.m. Not just because it's dark and people are indoors rather than enjoying the spring and summer evenings, but there is no clapping or clanging of pots anymore. I wish I could say it is because the pandemic is over, but it isn't. How we choose, as a nation, to work toward its end remains to be seen.

* * * * *

The prognosis for Covid-19 patients was not as dire as that of HIV/AIDS patients during my residency. Despite all the unknowns, all the anguish, and all the death, with Covid-19, we had hope that many of our patients would recover.

We celebrated those successes. Whenever a patient left the hospital, the staff lined the halls (all in masks) clapping and cheering as the patient rolled by in a wheelchair. One such "clap-out" was particularly memorable. Octavio Robles was a police officer from Union City, New Jersey. He had performed CPR on his mother, who had Covid-19. She did not survive, and shortly thereafter, he came down with the disease as well. He was very sick, requiring intubation shortly after arriving at Holy Name. His family was prepared for the fact that he, too, would probably not survive. But he did.

After two and a half weeks on a ventilator, Officer Robles was able to leave the hospital. He refused a wheelchair, insisting on walking out on his own. As he left the hospital he was greeted by what seemed like the entire police force of Union City, socially distanced and wearing masks, who had joined the hospital staff and his family for the clap-out. As Officer Robles walked away with his children, his fellow police officers followed behind.

Then one came back.

Nichelle Luster, the Union City Police Chief, wanted to address the hospital staff. She told us that the force had already lost one member to Covid-19, and that they had been all but certain that they would lose another. The officers – every one of them – would never forget what Holy Name had done for him, and for them, she said.

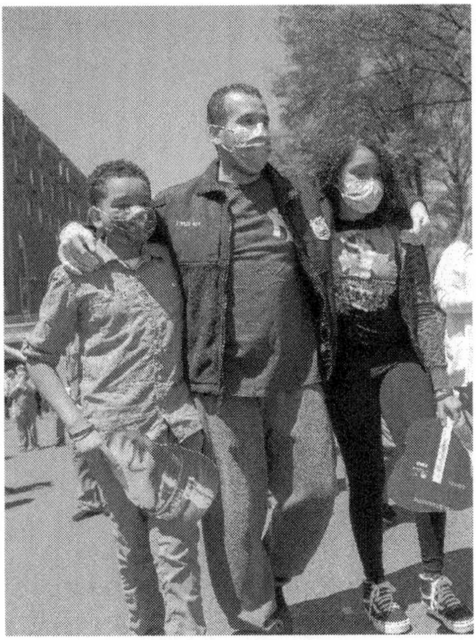

Officer Octavio Robles and his children as he walks out of Holy Name after successfully fighting Covid-19.

At Holy Name, we were particularly concerned about the mental health of our staff during this time. We were dealing not just with the emotional ups and downs of Covid-19, but also struggling with the fear of becoming infected ourselves or, far worse, infecting our loved ones. We had known the potential risks to ourselves when we entered the healthcare profession, but with Covid-19, our families were involuntary passengers along for the ride.

When I worked on the AIDS ward, everyone was worried about accidentally being stuck with a needle that had been used on an infected patient. One night, as I attempted to get a few hours of sleep in the on-call room, I was awakened by my beeper at 2:00 a.m. I cursed to myself; I had just settled down an hour earlier. Having gotten these late-night pages before on the AIDS ward, I knew it was most likely fevers – a common occurrence for our patients in the middle of the night, and a regular page after the nurses completed their rounds.

When this happened, the on-call intern would need to evaluate and culture the patients, looking for an opportunistic infection.

I sat on the side of the cot and tried to clear my head. My stomach twisted from the smell of old food that had been left out, and from the thought that I was likely going to be drawing blood cultures on multiple HIV-positive patients. I splashed some water on my face and headed to the nurses' station. The charge nurse was waiting for me, with a weary look on her face. "Mr. Johnson, Mr. Simon, and Mr. Rugerio are all spiking." Just as I had expected, "fever rounds."

I pulled out their charts and plopped down at the desk. I knew Johnson and Simon, two of my patients, well. Mr. Rugerio, however, was another intern's patient. After a brief review of the charts, I assessed each patient – they were all uncomfortable and had high fevers, but were clinically stable. It was the middle of the night, I was sleep-deprived, and I needed to stick each of these men with a needle twice in order to draw their blood, which would then be sent to the lab to look for an infection.

Sticking yourself with a needle was always a possibility when drawing blood and inserting IVs. It happened more commonly than you would think. And when you were exhausted due to interrupted and inadequate sleep, the risk was much greater.

I willed myself to stay focused and took all the blood samples with no incident.

Throughout my residency, I was never stuck with a needle. But several of my peers were. It created great anxiety and fear, though none of them contracted HIV/AIDS. The incidence of HIV infection from a needle stick was real, but low (needle sticks present a much higher risk for other diseases, such as viral hepatitis). The chance of being stuck with any needle today has been greatly reduced. Needles have been redesigned so that they draw back into their tube after use. In addition, we now have a cocktail of medications that is very effective in preventing HIV transmission to healthcare workers who are stuck with an infected needle.

Remarkably, the fear of getting infected and infecting loved ones felt even more intense in the time of Covid-19 than during the HIV/AIDS pandemic. Getting infected did not require a needle stick; it could happen from simply walking into a patient's room, if you were not adequately protected. Even though the chance of dying from Covid-19 was dramatically lower than a patient's chance of dying from HIV/AIDS in the '90s, the likelihood of getting infected – and then possibly infecting others – was much, much greater. This was a major stressor for staff, even with adequate PPE.

We did what we could to help reduce stress. First and foremost, we always prioritized staff safety when making decisions. We also created a Zen Den with massage chairs, free healthy snacks, and aromatherapy. We arranged for laundry drop-off and pick-up at the hospital, and even for a hair stylist to come in to provide haircuts – a real luxury when hair salons and barbershops, like many other businesses, were shuttered.

In addition, once or twice a day we would play an inspirational song on the loudspeakers throughout the hospital. Often these were performed by one of our nurses, Felicia Temple. Felicia was a finalist on *The Voice* a few years ago. She is incredibly talented and was actually on tour when Covid-19 hit. She left the tour and came back to work at the hospital because she knew that her nursing skills were desperately needed. Hearing her beautiful voice was a bright spot every day.

We also played a song every time we discharged a Covid-19 patient. We tried to pick a wide selection, from musical theater songs to Bruce Springsteen covers, but Mike often requested one of his favorite songs: an instrumental theme from the inspirational 1993 movie *Rudy*. *Rudy* is a biographical film about Daniel Ruettiger, a man who overcame great odds to play football for Notre Dame. It's a great movie, more about the people than the game.

*Rudy* was released in 1993, one year after I completed my residency. Looking back, as a young, naive intern just out of medical school, I was only superficially aware that we were in the midst of a pandemic that would ultimately claim more than 700,000 lives here in the U.S. I feel the same was true for most people about Covid-19, right up until it hit their communities. Then it became all too real.

I don't think it's possible to be fully prepared for the emotional challenges of a pandemic. However, my experience on the AIDS ward ingrained in me a strong awareness of the stress that comes with facing a new, horrible, and deadly disease. Dealing with the unknown, coping with the rapid increase in patients, and learning to accept the reality of the escalation in deaths is extremely taxing. The AIDS ward is where I learned to recognize and address my own stress, and now as a member of a leadership team, I do whatever I can to reduce the pressure on those working tirelessly for our Covid-19 patients.

**As of July 2020**

- 38 million people worldwide and 1.2 million in the US are living with HIV/AIDS.
- Only 67 percent of people with HIV/AIDS receive appropriate treatment.
- Because of Covid-19, 36 countries report disruption in treatment for HIV/AIDS patients.

CHAPTER SEVEN

# Stopping the Spread

*"60 days ago, this virus infection [Covid-19] was not even among the top 75 causes of death in the United States....For the last week and a half, it's been the number one cause of death day after day after day.*
*That's serious. This is not the flu."*

**Dr. Michael T. Osterholm**
Director, Center for Infectious Disease Research and Policy
University of Minnesota
April 17, 2020

In early March, I made a mistake. There was not yet talk about social distancing, and we thought our first Covid-19 patient was still a while off. In preparation, I called our medical staff together for a briefing on Covid-19, expecting about 50 physicians and nurses to show up. Much to my surprise, 500 people came to the meeting – not just nurses and physicians, but technicians, therapists, accounting staff, and even food service workers – an indication of the high level of interest and concern among staff.

During the meeting, Dr. Suraj Saggar, our Chief of Infectious Disease, discussed the current situation in China, Europe, and Washington State. He educated us about the virus itself, including what to look for in patients who might have Covid-19 and how to stay safe. Lastly, he reviewed Holy Name's plans to isolate Covid-19 patients.

However, what both Suraj and I had not thought of, and failed to mention, was that large gatherings in confined spaces – like the one we were holding – were dangerous. Only one doctor in the entire room of 500 people wore a mask, and he received several bewildered looks. Of course, we did not know that the very next day we would get not only our first confirmed Covid-19 patient, but six Covid-19 patients, or that we probably already had undiagnosed Covid-19 patients in the hospital, and possibly even staff who were already infected.

When we look back at the charts of patients who were in the hospital in January and February, there were definitely patients who, had they come in a few weeks later, would have been tested for and diagnosed with Covid-19. These patients were instead treated for flu, flu-like illnesses, or pneumonia. When we went from zero Covid-19 patients to six in one day, it was likely because we were all on high alert from the meeting the day before. With the symptoms fresh in our minds, we were looking for and able to identify these six patients the next day. The press soon learned that we had the greatest number of hospitalized Covid-19 patients in New Jersey, and they quickly identified us as the epicenter of the outbreak.

Eleven days later, Mike and I spoke at a press conference with our local congressman, several mayors, the Bergen County Executive, and a gaggle of reporters. We shared what we were seeing on the ground and gave our spiel about how our communities needed to do more to stop the virus from spreading throughout the community.

When we opened the floor to questions from the press, the first question we received was, "Is this conference safe?"

I think the reporter was asking if being close to Mike and me was dangerous, but the real danger for him was actually from the other reporters, who were closer to him than we were.

"Being close to us is not the concern," I replied. "We're six feet away from you. But your clustering together may put you at risk." I looked around at the other speakers behind the podium. "It's not great that we're all gathered around this podium and that we're not distancing. We should have set up a way to keep reporters six feet apart from each other and to not have everyone clustered together behind the microphone."

After that, I tried much harder to practice what I preached to help prevent the spread of the virus. I also became particularly aware of how members of the White House Task Force stood so close to each other while at the same time telling us all to socially distance. I realized relatively quickly the example we needed to set. Unfortunately, the same cannot be said for the White House.

* * * * *

When my mother cooked Thanksgiving dinner, she would bring out the fine tablecloth and the linen napkins, load the table with broccoli casserole, noodle kugel, and mashed turnips, bring out the turkey, and then step back and say, "That's a good spread." With Covid-19, a good spread is anything under one.

The spread of an infection is measured by its R(0) (pronounced "R-naught") factor. To put it simply, R(0) indicates how many people the typical person infects while they are infected. If each infected person infects exactly one other person (R(0) = 1), the amount of people sick with the virus remains constant over time. If the number goes above one (R(0) > 1), the number of infected people grows steadily, and if it drops below 1 (R(0) < 1), the number of sick people decreases. If the R(0) factor is zero, infections die out.

The R(0) factor for a pathogen can differ depending on the weather (for flu, it is higher in the winter and lower in the summer), and it varies by country as well (the R(0) factor for TB in the U.S. is less than 1, but as high as 4.3 in countries with a heavy TB burden).

Covid-19 is thought to have an R(0) of around 2.2. This number assumes that we do nothing to decrease the spread, and nothing to intentionally increase the spread, such as holding Covid-19 parties. This R(0) of 2.2 is higher than the typical flu. If left unchecked, Covid-19 will likely spread to nearly everyone across the country. In early March, we saw infections soar at an unbridled pace in the New York City area. The key health policy directive then was to drive the R(0) factor down as low as possible through the social practices that are now so well known: wearing masks, practicing social distancing, regular hand washing, and not touching our faces.

Different viruses spread in different ways, and we slowly learned – and are still learning – more and more about how Covid-19 spreads from one person to another.

Initially, the staff at Holy Name were not required to wear face masks at all times while they were in the hospital. We thought that since the patients were in negative pressure rooms, staff were not at risk to contract the disease outside of those rooms. We were also conscious of the potential shortage of PPE. So, while staff wore full protective gear when caring for Covid-19 patients, we did not have guidelines governing use of PPE in other parts of the hospital or in the hallways.

As it turned out, the greatest risk of getting infected at the hospital actually did not come from the patients; with full PPE, healthcare workers' risk of infection while caring for Covid-19 patients was relatively small. Not a single one of our critical care physicians, who were working day and night in our ICUs, became infected. The risk came instead from other members of the staff who might become infected while at home or in the community. When we realized that interactions with other staff members could increase the spread of Covid-19, we changed our policy to require mask-wearing throughout the entire hospital, specifically, N95 masks that could filter out aerosolized viral particles.

Prior to Covid-19, medical personnel typically wore masks to protect patients who were vulnerable – not themselves. For example, nurses and doctors wear masks in the OR when someone is undergoing surgery, or in the rooms of patients who have compromised immune systems.

When Covid-19 first arrived in the U.S., the general public was not told to wear masks. Masks were scarce, needed by hospital workers, and we thought they were unlikely to protect the wearer. Early on, that's what I told people – wearing a mask was an unnecessary precaution. But then we gained a better understanding of this virus; it is spread by asymptomatic people, and therefore wearing a mask is less about protecting you, and more protecting others (like grocery store workers and the gas station attendant) because you might have the disease and not know it. Our essential workers are truly essential. They are not able to stay home because we need them to help run society. So, we need to protect them as much as possible.

When health organizations and medical professionals began to recommend that every person wear a mask outside the home, not everyone took this recommendation seriously. My cynical side thinks that more people may have worn masks if they had been told it was to protect themselves, rather than to protect others.

Eventually, the science did prove that wearing a mask also provides a level of protection for the wearer in addition to protecting others. Consistent mask-wearing outside the house is now the current recommendation (though some still refuse to follow this guideline).

My favorite explanation of how masks work is a simple one: imagine a place where no one wears pants. If another person pees on you, you get wet. Now, if *you* put pants on and someone pees on you, you still get wet, but less so.

But if *the other person* wears pants and pees, you will be fine. Maybe a little graphic, but it makes the point. Wearing a mask provides you some protection, but, more importantly, wearing a mask helps prevent you from infecting others.

It amazes me that wearing or not wearing a mask has become political – and that many people resist wearing one because they feel it infringes on their freedom. Once Covid-19 was prevalent in our community, it simply made sense to put on a mask. In retrospect, we all should have been more open to wearing masks from the very beginning. In the New York metropolitan area, mask-wearing is likely the single most impactful thing we have done to decrease new infections. If we had embraced wearing masks sooner as a nation, and if there was not still resistance to this simple act, we could have significantly decreased the Covid-19 infection and mortality rates.

We can't deny that the medical community gave poor advice regarding masks at the start of the pandemic. There's no shame in admitting we made a mistake, especially if we learn from that mistake and then apply what we learned, as we have done in this situation. What is shameful, however, is the deliberate and intentional spread of misinformation, which can take on a life of its own and prove disastrous in a pandemic.

Wearing a mask does not impede oxygen flow to the brain. Nor does it increase the likelihood of spreading the disease. Both of these claims gained traction early in the pandemic, and are still parroted by anti-maskers today. Some anti-maskers also claim that stores and other establishments that require masks violate a legal right – also untrue. Requirements that shoppers wear a mask are no more an infringement on freedom than are requirements that shoppers wear a shirt and shoes.

I like to compare wearing a mask with smoking. Until relatively recently, smoking was unregulated. Nonsmokers may not have been happy to breathe in secondhand smoke in restaurants or planes, but it was thought to be nothing more than a nuisance. Once clear scientific evidence showed that breathing in secondhand smoke was harmful, the laws changed. It is unfair and, frankly, wrong to allow innocent bystanders to be harmed by the actions of others. That is why you cannot smoke in an indoor public space, and that is why you should wear a mask during a pandemic.

Another way to reduce Covid-19's R(0) factor is through social distancing. In the extreme, if you interact with no one (the ultimate in social distancing), your risk of catching or spreading the disease is zero. Common wisdom is that the acceptable "safe" distance is six feet apart from one another. As one person explained it to me, always stay one moose length away (though it appears that a moose is closer to eight feet long, so perhaps that person was extra cautious).

What is the magic in six feet? It is the distance where, in most cases, droplets generated from breathing, talking, and laughing will have dropped to the ground. Coughing, or worse yet, sneezing, sends the droplets further. But if the virus is aerosolized (meaning it lingers in the air), six feet is woefully inadequate.

Take, for example, a professor at a university.

If the university erects a plexiglass barrier that allows the students (socially distanced six feet apart from each other) to see and hear the professor, the plexiglass will effectively stop any droplets that she emits from reaching the students. But if that professor is wearing perfume and air is circulating so that the students can get a whiff of the scent, then the plexiglass is not protecting them from the aerosolized perfume – or an aerosolized virus. If there is a virus circulating in the air, the professor could still infect the students, or the students could infect the professor and each other.

As discussed, there is still some debate over whether Covid-19 spreads via droplets or aerosols. Holy Name treats the disease as though it is spread by both (hence the importance of negative pressure rooms and ISO-pods for all Covid-19 or suspected Covid-19 patients).

When a virus is aerosolized, social distancing is more effective outside, where the virus can dissipate with natural airflow. A study from Japan has concluded that someone exposed to Covid-19 indoors is 19 times more likely to be infected than when exposed in the same way outdoors. And in China, a study of 1,000 infected people investigated how they were exposed and found only one situation in which outdoor transmission occurred, infecting two patients. However, you should still wear masks and practice social distancing even when outside.

Many people thought at first that the Covid-19 infection operated like a switch. If you came in contact with the virus, it would switch on, and you were immediately infected. That is not how it works.

When your body is exposed to a virus, your immune system can fight off a certain, small level of virus. But if you are exposed to a large amount of the virus – either through a large event (like a sneeze) or through sustained exposure to smaller amounts (like spending several hours in a room with someone infected with Covid-19) – your immune system can be overwhelmed. Once this happens, you get infected. The amount of virus that you are exposed to (called the viral dose) may also play a role in how sick you actually get. Some people may get infected when exposed to a small viral dose, but that infection may be less severe than if that person had experienced a larger viral dose. If you are exposed to Covid-19, wearing a mask will decrease the amount of virus that enters your system, decreasing your risk of infection and the likelihood that you will experience a severe illness.

In early March, as concern over the virus's spread began to grow within the local communities, I attended a meeting with members of the town of Oradell's Covid-19 Task Force. Among other things, the task force wanted to know if they should close the schools and how they should support their EMT professionals. I advised them to close the schools, or to at least begin to prepare for closing; closings were inevitable, so they would be ahead of the curve (though even I did not think they would stay closed for the remainder of the year).

At the time, this was a radical recommendation. I certainly got my share of questioning looks. I also recommended that they get PPE for their EMT squad and require its use to minimize the risk of spreading infections. Finally, I told them to be prepared to close down the town infrastructure – the library, the Department of Public Works, and the town hall. The leader of the task force nodded, but looked grim.

I had a similar meeting with an official from the State Department of Health and the heads of the Orthodox Jewish communities in Teaneck and neighboring towns. After the State official told them that he could not make a recommendation one way or the other about closing the schools and the temples, I told them that based on what I was seeing at the hospital and the known infectivity of this virus, they should close down. I was concerned with how quickly the virus had spread in the Orthodox Jewish communities in New York State, and knew that it had spread to the Orthodox Jewish communities in Teaneck. After heated debate, the Jewish schools and temples closed the next day. I believe this action saved lives. With a virus that had an R(0) of 2.2, staying open an extra week likely would have had a significant impact on the total number of people infected.

To reduce the spread of the virus within the hospital, we replaced our daily in-person meetings with video chats. These meetings were vital for our core group of managers who met throughout the day to discuss how to meet the needs of our patients over the next 24 hours – how many beds to convert, how we were doing with PPE, any staffing concerns, and whatever else arose that day.

When someone suggested that it would be nice if we could spend part of our 16-plus hour days getting some fresh air, we decided to move our end-of-day meeting outside. So every day at 5 p.m. (weather permitting), we gathered outside in a large circle in the once-bustling parking lot, which was now for the most part empty of cars. We stood six feet apart, without masks, which were not yet mandated for general use.

One of our first socially distanced outside meetings. Later, we would require attendees to wear masks.

Fear of how easily the virus could spread impacted our construction team at the hospital as well. While the contractors did not come into contact with Covid-19 patients, they were working 18 hours a day converting rooms. We quickly decided to house them in nearby hospital-owned residences. Some of the team lived 30 or 40 miles away, and we couldn't ask them to drive home at midnight, only to drive back for a 6 a.m. start the next morning. We expected this

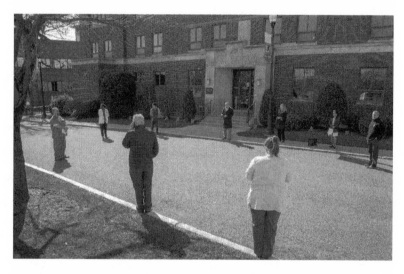

temporary housing situation would last a few days; it lasted nearly five weeks.

When the workers told their spouses that they would be staying in Teaneck, their spouses assumed it was because they were potentially infectious. In truth, the construction crew presented no higher a risk of infection than the rest of the hospital staff.

But when the crews finally completed the construction and were ready to return home, their spouses didn't want them. They were afraid of being infected by people who had spent weeks working around the clock in a hospital called the "Covid Epicenter."

The workers didn't know what to do. That afternoon, Mike stopped by my office. "Adam, I need you to call the construction crew's families."

I stood up from my desk so I could better see Mike, who remained outside my open door. "Why me?" I asked.

"You're the one doing most of the media," he said. "They'll trust you."

It was true that I had become the public face of the hospital, appearing on news shows and doing press calls with our congressman. But I didn't think that qualified me to intervene in our employees' marriages. I picked up the phone anyway, calling Steve's wife first, since he had overseen the construction.

When she picked up the phone, I assured her that the workers had never done construction around infected patients. I explained the concept of negative pressure rooms, and told her that all staff who came in contact with Covid-19 patients wore PPE. Lastly, I explained that if she had gone to the grocery store, where she may have been exposed to the disease, she presented just as much of a risk to Steve as he presented to her.

She finally said that Steve could come home that night, and the rest of the crew's spouses eventually agreed. None of the construction workers became infected.

* * * * *

Ultimately, all activity beyond complete isolation brings some risk. Relatives and friends often ask me, “Can I do this?” or “Can I do that?” “Can I go to the post office?” “Can I have a game night with just a few people?” “Can I go to a bachelor party?” There is rarely a definitive answer. Everything falls somewhere on a spectrum. There is little risk of contracting Covid-19 while wearing a mask and taking a walk in the park with your spouse. On the other hand, going to an indoor wedding with 250 guests where there is minimal mask wearing presents a high risk.

In deciding what you should or shouldn’t do, you need to evaluate the risk (taking into account your own health condition), the availability of safer alternatives, and how much risk you are comfortable taking (for yourself, and for those you regularly come in contact with).

This doesn’t just apply to all of us as individuals. We need to have this same mindset as a society. Until we have an effective, safe, and widespread vaccine and improved therapeutics, individuals and society as a whole will have to constantly balance the risk of moving the R(0) factor up with the benefits of introducing more risk into our lives and attempting to return to some semblance of normalcy.

**Early Super-Spreader Events**

- **February 26**, Boston, Massachusetts: Ninety attendees are infected at a Biogen conference. More than 20,000 cases have since been directly or indirectly linked to attendees, including cases in Virginia, North Carolina, Texas, Australia, Sweden, and Slovakia.
- **February 27**, Westchester, New York: A man attends a bat mitzvah, religious services, and a birthday party; 170 cases are later linked to this original spreader.
- **Late February**, Chicago, Illinois: One individual who was infected at a funeral passes Covid-19 on to seven others at a birthday party, one of whom passed it on to 16 people at a church service. In total, three died.
- **March 5**, Westport, Connecticut: Forty people attend a birthday party, 20 become infected and then return home to places such as New York City and South Africa.

CHAPTER EIGHT

# The Search for PPE

***Hawkeye**: What's this?*

***Radar**: Weekend passes for the raffle.*

***Hawkeye**: When did he sign these?*

***Radar**: When he thought he was ordering a ton of ice cream. Fudge ripple.*

**From TV Series *M*A*S*H***
Season 1, Episode 1 (Pilot)
Airdate – September 17, 1972

My favorite character on the '70s TV series *M*A*S*H* was Radar O'Reilly. As company clerk of the MASH (Mobile Army Surgical Hospital) unit, Radar was responsible for procuring everything from scalpels to ladies' lingerie, and he was particularly good at finding smart ways to get items that were in short supply. He didn't break the rules, but he definitely bent them.

Holy Name's Radar is Don Ecker, a tall, thin man who never had a hair out of place even in the midst of the pandemic, and who always chooses the exact right socks for the outfit or the occasion. Even before the first confirmed Covid-19 case hit our shores, the normal supply routes for PPE, coming mostly out of China, had dried up. This presented a hopefully once in a lifetime challenge for Don, our Director of Supply Chain.

Just as Radar kept things running as smoothly as possible in a time of war, Don was essential to Holy Name's operations as we struggled to care for our patients and keep our staff safe. Every day, Don would listen to the medical and nursing staff describe what was needed for their patients and for themselves, and after asking a few key follow-up questions so he could prioritize his list, Don would hit the phones.

Don conducted an endless hunt for masks, gowns, gloves, goggles, and ventilators. In addition to calling his regular contacts and suppliers, Don would also follow up on the many emails I and other staff members received every day offering much needed medical supplies available for purchase. Ninety percent of these turned out to be false leads, but Don pursued every one of them to uncover the handful that would make a critical difference.

During the early months of the pandemic, Don got masks from veterinarians, construction workers (who use N95 masks to protect against dust and chemicals), people in the local community who dropped them off at the hospital in handfuls (extras they had lying around the garage), the federal stockpile, and a growing list of suppliers who had masks available – for a price.

N95 masks that had sold for 99 cents or less before Covid-19, were now selling for $3 to $5. Vendors who had a large supply were able to turn a good profit. While some might say it was criminal to profit from other people's struggles, or at the very least that it was unethical, this didn't stop people from trying to line their pockets during the pandemic. Many businesses and individuals reaped tremendous profits during the pandemic by selling products to hospitals at inflated prices.

Some reported "mask sellers" were less credible than others. One man called the hospital and said he had a ship full of N95 masks sitting in international waters off the coast of New Jersey. As we did with all leads, we followed up. He wanted money up front. We suggested meeting at the Jersey Shore to see the supply firsthand. He balked, and then disappeared.

Masks are a key component in the fight against the spread of infection.

Different types of masks serve different purposes. Surgical masks are primarily used to prevent the spread of germs from hospital staff to a patient. They differ from N95 masks, which are primarily designed to keep the wearer safe. In normal times, a hospital goes through many more surgical masks than N95 masks.

An N95 mask prevents 95 percent of particles from passing through the mask. Healthcare professionals wear this type of mask when we are concerned about patients who might infect us – particularly with an infection that is aerosolized, such as TB, measles, Ebola, chickenpox, or Covid-19. N100 masks, which filter out 99.7 percent of airborne particles, are typically used in industrial settings and can be washed and reused as long as their filters are replaced regularly. These masks tend to make breathing difficult and are not routinely used in healthcare.

N95 masks must fit correctly to be effective. Once a year, every clinical member of our staff is fitted for an N95 mask. The clinician puts on an N95 mask, and then a hood is slipped over their head. A chemical is sprayed into the hood, and if the individual can smell the sweet spray, the mask is not a good fit. The clinician repeats the process with different sizes until they find the right fit.

The most effective "mask" is not a mask at all. It's called a Powered Air Purifying Respirator (PAPR), and it fits entirely over your head. It looks like one of those old deep-sea diving helmets with a glass face and an air tube leading to the surface. It has a mechanism that sucks in contaminated air from the room, draws it through a filter, and purifies it. N95 masks are effective, but PAPRs are nearly foolproof. They are expensive and, in the past, each hospital only ever needed a few at one time. Typically, Holy Name has about five of them on hand. When Covid-19 hit, we tried to get more, but couldn't.

In March, a friend's brother reached out to me and told me he had access to a large supply of PAPRs. They were made overseas, he said, and if we were interested, he would donate them to the hospital. Excited, I asked him to ship me one so that my team could evaluate its effectiveness. It sounded like this might be a solution to our problem, but Don was skeptical. When the PAPR arrived, Don brought it to our emergency preparedness team. He came back later that day – the PAPRs were a no-go. We had known in advance that they were not Food and Drug Administration (FDA)-approved – honestly, that might not have stopped us from using them if they were otherwise safe. But these PAPRs did not have an adequate air seal and would have exposed the wearer to the virus. I contacted my friend's brother and told him the bad news; he was apologetic, and sounded even more frustrated than I was.

Our limited number of PAPRs led to some heated discussions about who should use them. Anesthesiologists, who control patient pain by inducing and monitoring sedation during surgery, work closest to the patient's mouth. During the pandemic, they worked in our ICUs, assisting with daily patient management. The anesthesiologists argued that they experienced the highest risk due to their proximity to the patient's airway, so they should get the few PAPRs we had.

Others argued that the risk to the anesthesiologists was no greater than the risk to the nurses and technicians who were just a few inches further away from the patient's mouth. In the end, the PAPRs went to a few caregivers who could not shave their beards for religious reasons (facial hair lowers N95 effectiveness) and to the anesthesiologists.

While this decision felt somewhat arbitrary, few decisions during Covid-19 were clear cut. We did not always have time to establish a well-reasoned set of criteria upon which to base decisions. We went with our gut and moved on.

* * * * *

The quality of a mask matters. Masks were the frontline defense for our staff, and it was Don and the rest of his team's responsibility to not only make sure we had an adequate supply of masks, but to ensure that the masks were safe and effective.

We developed a three-tiered inspection system to ensure the quality of masks we received from new, and therefore unvetted, sources. First, our Manager of Infection Control, Ashley Blanchard, did an initial review. She checked the masks' materials, shape, and certifications. If they passed her examination, they went into use. But if Ashley wasn't satisfied, she brought the masks to an infection control physician and Don, the next tier in our system. They would further examine the masks to determine if they were safe to use. If they disagreed with each other or were still on the fence, they would bring the masks to me.

We took this process very seriously. Our staff was working in dangerous circumstances with a lot of unknowns, and having the right PPE didn't just ensure their safety, but also gave them peace of mind.

Early on, we received a supply of 7,000 N95 masks from the national stockpile, a supply of medical items that the government can provide to supplement hospitals during public health emergencies. Mike had been in constant contact with New Jersey Governor Phil Murphy, explaining to him how hard we had been hit and how desperately we needed PPE. Murphy delivered: we were one of the first hospitals to receive our share of masks from the government. He called us one day to let us know the masks were coming, although he didn't know when or how. One early morning, we simply discovered a large pallet of boxes on our loading dock.

Like all disposable medical supplies, the masks were marked with an expiration date – which had already come and gone. At first, we weren't worried;

a few weeks prior, the FDA had announced that masks from the federal stockpile were safe to use, regardless of their expiration date.

Unfortunately, this was not the case. When we tested the masks, several of them ripped apart – surely not something you want to happen when you are dealing with this type of infection. I am not sure if the poor performance was related to the quality or the age of the masks, but either way, we didn't want to risk a mask tearing while a staff member was in a Covid-19 room. We continued to use other, safer masks instead, and put the federal stockpile masks in storage, just in case; if the situation became desperate, they might be better than nothing. To this day, we have not used them.

Quality-control issues continued to be a headache throughout the pandemic. One week, we received 500 defective masks from one of our usual suppliers. Word got out that we had been a victim of fraud, and a half dozen reporters called Holy Name looking for a story where there wasn't one; the supplier took the masks back without a problem and replaced them with high-quality N95s. However, I lost a few hours that I didn't really have to spare convincing reporters that there was no newsworthy story here.

Although we were having so much trouble finding masks, one day I returned home to my Manhattan apartment to find that our building doorman was wearing an N95 mask. The management firm had given him and the other doormen a small supply, probably ones the building had had on hand for maintenance work. I didn't begrudge the building staff their masks; hundreds of people passed by the doormen every day, a risk that certainly justified masks. But I was a little jealous. Imagine my surprise when I arrived at my apartment door to find a box of masks that had been dropped on our welcome mat. I had no idea where they had come from, but I gladly passed them on to Don. I later learned one of my neighbors had provided the masks because she knew I was a healthcare worker. We had never – and still have not – met, but I was extremely grateful.

Thankfully, we never ran out of masks ay Holy Name. It provided us some sense of relief knowing we were doing everything we could to protect our staff. But just as important as having a mask to wear was knowing how to safely put it on and take it off to reduce the chance of infection.

We had learned during our preparation for Ebola that the technique used for donning and doffing (formal words for putting on and taking off) of PPE mattered. At that time, the CDC had published guidelines explaining how to don and doff PPE. We wanted to test those guidelines ourselves, so, facing the potential of an Ebola epidemic in 2014, we headed to the Simulation Center.

We set up a simulated exam room with an actor pretending to be an Ebola patient. To simulate body fluids, we applied red paint to the patient's body. The staff member attending the patient would don PPE according to CDC guidelines outside the room, then go in to "attend" to the patient. After exiting the room, the staff member would doff the PPE, again, following CDC guidelines.

After our first test, we were dismayed to see red paint on the doctor who had participated in the simulation – on her neck, face, and wrists. If the patient had actually had Ebola, the doctor would have been infected.

We realized that CDC guidelines, which identified the "correct" PPE to wear when treating Ebola patients, were wholly inadequate. We re-ran the simulation with total body Kevlar suits with hoods and discovered that they actually protected staff – no red paint. Not long after we uncovered this issue, the CDC also changed their guidelines to full body suits for Ebola protection.

The key takeaways from this exercise? Do not blindly accept guidelines, especially when working with a new disease.

Now faced with Covid-19, we applied what we had learned during our Ebola simulations to develop our PPE procedures for this new virus. While both diseases are highly contagious, Ebola is far more deadly than Covid-19. Both diseases have an R(0) factor of about 2, but Ebola's R(0) factor is only that low because it kills its victims so quickly that they are not able to infect many other people, and because it is only spread through bodily fluid, not aerosols.

Ebola has a 90 percent mortality rate, exponentially higher than Covid-19's. It can also enter the body through microscopic tears in the skin. This combination of deadliness and high risk of transmission warranted extreme precautions.

Covid-19, while dangerous, has a significantly lower mortality rate than Ebola and typically only spreads via inhalation. When a healthcare worker gets Covid-19 on their hands (which should not happen if they're wearing gloves), it does not pose an imminent risk as long as the worker does not touch their face and quickly washes their hands. The differences between Ebola and Covid-19 meant that the PPE that had been inadequate for dealing with Ebola patients – masks, gloves, and gowns – provided sufficient protection to staff members working with Covid-19 patients.

I saw our own nurses, doctors, and technicians stretched to the limit while caring for our Covid-19 patients. I can't imagine having them do so without adequate PPE. Nevertheless, there are healthcare workers in the U.S. who continued to work as the rest of society hunkered down, and who needlessly fell ill because there was not enough PPE available. This is a national disgrace.

Early on, we calculated roughly how many masks we would need. We decided that even with Don's herculean efforts, we could not meet the 1,500-3,000 estimated masks we would need each day. We thought long and hard about our processes and how we could conserve PPE without endangering staff or patients. At the beginning of the pandemic, standard practice was for staff to put on a fresh N95 mask every time they saw a different patient. We soon realized that wasn't sustainable, so we adjusted our protocols. We decided that staff should wear an N95 mask when interacting with Covid-19 patients, and then a surgical mask over it to protect the outside of the N95. Staff changed the outer surgical mask (of which we had an adequate but not unlimited supply) after each patient, but kept the N95 on as long as they were working with Covid-19 patients. When the staff member was done caring for Covid-19 patients, they would remove their surgical mask and N95 and place the N95 in a sealed plastic bag.

These N95 masks, as well as all face shields and goggles, were then treated with UV light and put in storage in case they were needed in the future. Several studies have shown that UV light eliminates viruses and bacteria on the outside of protective gear. While we were concerned that the intensity of UV light might undermine the integrity of the masks, we were confident that it would kill any Covid-19 on the masks. And we knew that if only treated once, the masks would maintain their integrity. (Goggles, since they are made of plastic, can be treated with UV light multiple times without risking damage.) We haven't yet had to use these UV-treated N95 masks, but like the masks we received from the federal stockpile, we have them ready to go should we ever need them.

To further minimize the risk our staff faced, we developed a simple but thorough procedure for donning and doffing PPE:

1. Put on a clean N95 mask.
2. Apply a clean surgical mask over the N95.
3. After caring for a Covid-19 patient, remove the surgical mask by the straps and dispose, being careful not to touch the front of either the

surgical mask or the N95.

4. Put on a fresh surgical mask before caring for the next Covid-19 patient, again being careful not to touch the front of the N95.
5. Repeat Step 4 between every Covid-19 patient.
6. When done caring for Covid-19 patients (taking a break, going to nurses' station to document in the medical record, etc.), remove the surgical mask as described above and then remove the N95 by the straps, being careful not to touch the front of the mask. Place the N95 in a plastic bag to be processed for UV decontamination and storage.
7. Remove and dispose of gloves in a biohazard receptacle.
8. Every time any mask is removed, staff must wash hands and apply fresh gloves. Staff must also wash hands every time gloves are removed.

If this sounds tedious, that's because it was. But it was also necessary.

Each staff member watched a mandatory video demonstrating this procedure and explaining the proper way to take off and roll a gown, making sure that the potentially infected area is always on the inside and the clean side of the gown on the outside. Staff were diligent in following these instructions and reminding co-workers to comply.

Some hospitals that were not able to obtain an adequate supply of masks instructed staff members to use the same N95 throughout the day, or sometimes even longer. Other hospitals that did not have enough N95 masks had their staff use surgical masks instead. During the pandemic, a young family friend was in her internship at a Seattle hospital where doctors and nurses mostly wore surgical masks. During a code blue, the charge nurse would bring out a bucket of fresh N95 masks for members of the code team to wear during the code, but staff did not normally wear N95s when interacting with Covid-19 patients.

We did not want staff to re-use previously worn N95 masks, which would likely have live virus on their outsides. If staff had to re-use masks, where would the potentially-infectious masks be stored? It was safer to dispose of used masks immediately, so we instructed our staff to never re-use their N95 masks. This made it even more essential to have a steady and sufficient supply of PPE.

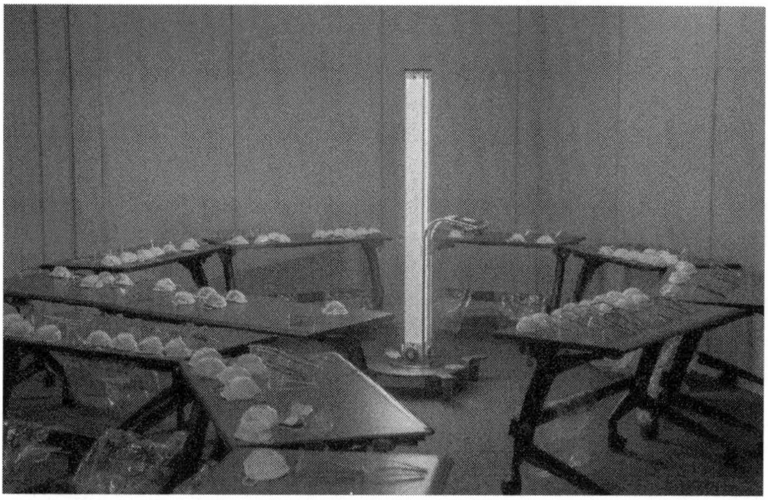

We used UV lights to disinfect PPE, which was then stored for possible future use.

The few times we actually had masks to spare, we shared them with other nearby hospitals. When Don sent some to The Valley Hospital, in neighboring Ridgewood, New Jersey, they returned the favor by providing us with a pandemic ventilator, a basic ventilator that lacked some of the bells and whistles most ventilators had, but that could still be used to provide emergency oxygen to patients. In general, the level of inter-hospital cooperation at this time was remarkable. For the first time in my 15 years as a hospital administrator, I saw hospitals working together rather than working against each other. It was honestly a nice break from the constant competition that is an unfortunate reality in healthcare today. This cooperation resulted in better care for all our patients, and also helped keep staff safe.

Because he was so good at it, Don found himself procuring masks not only for Holy Name, but for other hospitals as well. One day, after receiving yet another call from a local hospital desperately in need of masks, Don asked if he could share his supplier list with their procurement staff. Of course, I said yes.

When Don called his counterpart to share his list, the other hospital wouldn't take it. According to their materials manager, they could not receive masks directly from vendors who were not approved – but it was okay to accept them if we acted as the middleman. This didn't really make sense to us; even if we were the direct supplier to this hospital, the masks we had procured and provided were still coming from "unapproved" vendors. But we agreed to supply the masks to the other hospital ourselves to ensure their staff did not run out of PPE. In this time of crisis, we were okay with bending some rules, even if others were less willing to do so.

In addition to figuring out how to keep enough masks on hand, we also needed to maintain an adequate supply of gowns. Initially, our nurses used disposable gowns, the norm in today's hospitals. At the peak of the pandemic, each nurse went through 15-20 gowns every shift, and the hospital used and disposed of 2,500 gowns per day. We were dangerously close to running out.

However, we also had a supply of reusable cloth gowns leftover from the days before disposable gowns became the standard. On one of our daily strategy calls, with a shortage of disposable gowns looming, Don suggested that we shift to using the cloth gowns. There was only one problem: no laundry service had the capacity to wash several thousand gowns nightly and deliver them to the hospital the following morning.

Dave Van Bever, who oversees housekeeping, came to the rescue. He reached out to the laundry facility in Maryland that delivers fresh laundry (sheets and patient gowns) to us weekly. When Dave asked if they could also launder the cloth gowns for our staff, they told us yes, their washing machines could handle the extra volume Monday through Friday. But they wouldn't be able to pick up and deliver the gowns daily. Instead, we recruited four of our staff who had transported patients for elective surgeries prior to Covid-19 to be gown transporters. Every day, two of them made the eight-hour round trip to Maryland to drop off half our gowns, dirty from a day's use, and pick up the other half of newly-cleaned gowns.

Around 7 p.m. each evening, they arrived back at the hospital, where a team of 30 would spend the next two to three hours sorting and preparing the gowns for use. Our limited supply of disposable gowns was just enough to get us through Saturday and Sunday when the laundry facility was closed.

It turned out that the nursing staff greatly preferred the reusable gowns to the disposable ones. They were more comfortable, and the nurses felt like the cloth gowns provided better protection. Post-Covid-19, Holy Name will be sticking with the reusable gowns – though we will no longer need the daily runs to Maryland.

We also dealt with a shortage of ventilators. Hospitals strive for product consistency – it improves safety. All our ventilators at Holy Name are usually the same. That way, staff only need to learn one operating process, and parts can be easily exchanged between one machine and another.

In the midst of Covid-19, however, we had a hodgepodge of ventilators. Don would get them wherever he could, however he could, and in whatever quantity he could, and he would do whatever was necessary to get them up and running.

One day he got six machines from the Bronx that had been used as eaching units. Four were good to go, two needed to be refurbished. The cost for he six was $100,000, a reasonable price. Another day, Don tracked down five units in Hartford, Connecticut, from a medical equipment refurbisher who would rent them to us for six months for a total of $12,000, also a reasonable price.

Every time he located a new set of ventilators, Don hopped in a truck and went and got them. Prior to Covid-19, we had 14 ventilators at the hospital, and usually no more than six or seven patients who needed them.

I can't talk about ventilators without mentioning Roy Morris. Have you ever tried the "Florida Man" game? It's a game that pokes gentle fun at the state of Florida, which is notorious for having more than its fair share of colorful and front-page worthy characters. Search your birthday and the words "Florida man" in Google, and see what headline comes up – and there is a headline for everything. For example, when you Google "Florida Man" and Eileen's birthday, August 10, you'll find that her "Florida Man" headline is *Florida Man Arrested for DUI Says He Smoked Pot to Prepare for Jesus to Return.* (My "Florida Man" headline is less fit-for-print, but my birthday is January 8, if you want to look it up yourself.)

Well, Holy Name had an "Arkansas Man" headline: *Arkansas Man Shows up in Parking Lot to Fix Ventilators*. Okay, not as fun as *Florida Man Finds Alligator Relaxing in Jacuzzi* or *Florida Man Arrested for Brawling While Wearing an Easter Bunny Suit* or, my favorite, *Florida Man Fights Tree, Loses*, but still, an important story to us.

One day, after seeing a story about Holy Name, a vendor contacted us about someone who might be able to help us with our ventilator shortage – Roy Morris.

Roy is a biomedical engineer who has spent much of his career working both in academic medical centers and private industry, but his real passion is the work he does for International Children's Heart Foundation (ICHF). ICHF provides much needed cardiac surgery to children in developing countries. Roy works with hospitals around the United States and Canada collecting donated medical equipment such as ventilators, lasers, and intra-aortic balloon pumps. He refurbishes and re-certifies them so that they can be used all over the world. After Roy came to our attention, Don reached out to him and Roy offered to donate a few refurbished ventilators.

During that conversation, Don realized that Roy would be invaluable to Holy Name. Don easily convinced Roy to bring the ventilators to Holy Name himself so that he could examine the rest of our ventilator stock, which was not yet fully operational even with Don's hard work. On April 2, Roy and his son Samuel hopped in an RV and started the drive from Arkansas to New Jersey. They started the trip with 10 ventilators and picked up an additional six on the way north.

Roy and Samuel lived in our parking lot for a month. They became vital members of our team, lending a hand wherever they could, which included helping to make our new ICU beds operational. Most evenings, after a long, hard day, Roy and Samuel could be found sitting outside their RV in our parking lot sharing a meal with Mike or our security team.

After their time with us, Roy and Samuel headed back to Arkansas and self-quarantined for the necessary two weeks before Roy returned to his amazing work with ICHF. If you go to ICHF's website, you can learn more about Roy and the organization.

Even with Don and Roy's efforts, we didn't have enough ventilators. So we made adjustments to our continuous positive airway pressure (CPAP) machines (normally used for treating sleep apnea), which allowed us to use them as ventilators. Additionally, we were able to use anesthesia machines as short-term ventilators when absolutely necessary. We only resorted to these options a few times while we were waiting to secure other equipment, but they worked as temporary fixes.

Despite all of this, we worried that the demand for ventilators might exceed our supply. Finally, we turned to an idea we had only seen in reports and YouTube videos: the use of one ventilator for two or more patients. There were several short articles in the medical literature about doing this, but I was not aware of a hospital actually attempting this in a clinical setting.

Don, working with the anesthesiologists and the respiratory therapists, gathered a collection of parts and began to tinker in our Simulation Center. It was challenging.

Ventilators are machines that provide oxygen to patients who are unable to breathe on their own. In layman's terms, they can control how much oxygen a patient gets, how often and how quickly they get it, and the pressure at which the oxygen is administered. These settings are different for every patient and for every clinical situation. One patient might need oxygen at 10 breaths a second at 5 centimeters of water (the pressure), while another might need it at 16 breaths a second at 10 centimeters of water. This is a simple example, but the possibilities of different settings are endless.

By hooking a second tube up to a ventilator, we were able to put two mannequins on one machine in the Simulation Center. But we quickly realized that unless both patients were of the same build and weight and their lungs were being impacted in the same manner, we could not optimize the ventilator settings for both patients. Placing two patients on one ventilator would create a balancing act; we would have to either use suboptimal settings for both patients, or optimal settings for one and even worse settings for the other. Ultimately, we abandoned this approach. It wasn't practical to spend more time and resources on a theory that might never work in practice when we could instead focus on sourcing ventilators.

For four weeks, we spent every afternoon counting patients, evaluating who would need a ventilator and attempting to determine which patients currently on ventilators might not make it through the night – a tough reality. We also estimated how many patients might arrive the next day and have to be placed on ventilators immediately. Eventually, we had 84 ventilators, 28 of them from the national stockpile (these were not in working order when they arrived, but Don and his team fixed them). At our peak, we had 45 patients on ventilators.

We even created the position of "Ventilator Czar," a role filled by Ron White, a colo-rectal surgeon and lawyer who also heads our risk management department. Ron tracked all information related to ventilators and reported to the team at least daily. Every day, I was concerned that we were going to run out of ventilators, but thanks to Don and his team, we never did.

We also named a "Mask Czar," Randy Tartacoff, the physician co-director of our ED. He was in charge of everything masks – tracking how many we used, how many we needed, and what types and how many we currently had. Randy made sure Don knew both our short-term (tomorrow) and long-term (next few days to a week) needs.

Neither Ron nor Randy had expected to oversee emergency supply inventories when they joined Holy Name, but both were passionate about their new roles. They understood how important ventilators and masks were to saving lives and to the safety of the Holy Name staff.

* * * * *

When I stumble upon an episode of *M*A*S*H* as I flip through the channels at home, trying to get my mind off of work for a few minutes, I always leave it on. It is one of my favorite television shows. The acting is great, the stories are hilarious, and there is often an important message. After living through this pandemic, its appeal has grown even further. It portrays a group of dedicated healthcare professionals working together in an impossible situation. Those characters were in the midst of a war, and in a sense, during Covid-19, so were we.

**PPE Use at Holy Name**
**March 2020-July 2020**

- Gloves: 2,700,000
- N95 Masks: 186,000
- Surgical Masks: 846,000
- Goggles: 25,000

CHAPTER NINE

# Wishing for a Silver Bullet

*"I think what worries me is that people say, 'I've got a vaccine, I'm good,' as if we just sprinkled some magic powder across the land that means they don't need to wear a mask and can engage in high risk activity."*

**Dr. Paul Offit**
Director, Vaccine Education Center
Children's Hospital of Philadelphia

I don't enjoy bursting bubbles, but as a doctor, I sometimes have to deliver bad news. I believe being open and honest is almost always the best path forward – but that is not always easy to practice in the medical world. So, here goes: it is unlikely that a vaccine will be the silver bullet we are all hoping for. There, I said it. Now, let's hope I am wrong, but understand why I feel this way.

There are several big hurdles we need to overcome if a vaccine is to allow us to return to normal:

**1. Historically, vaccines take time to develop.**

It took four years to develop the mumps vaccine – the fastest effective vaccine ever developed. In 1963, Dr. Maurice Hilleman took a swab of his infected 5-year-old daughter's throat and brought it into work to help him develop a vaccine. Not good science by today's standards, but four years later, this swab had led to an effective vaccine.

Medicine has advanced a great deal since the 1960s, and the worldwide effort to develop a Covid-19 vaccine seems to be on the verge of success, which is remarkable considering that scientists have been working on a vaccine for HIV for close to 40 years to no avail. That virus mutates frequently, changing in a way that makes vaccine development very challenging. There is also no natural immunity to HIV, and without treatment, it is nearly 100 percent fatal. Even the human body has not figured out how to fight HIV, so there is no biological model that scientists can mimic in their search for a vaccine.

It seems likely that mRNA technology, a recent development in cancer treatment and vaccine research, has surpassed all expectations in the quest to develop a Covid-19 vaccine. As of the publishing of this book, the FDA seems poised to grant emergency access for two vaccines by the end of 2020. However, it is extremely important that the FDA follow their rigorous processes to assure the effectiveness and safety of these vaccines. All evidence suggests they will.

**2. The vaccine needs to be effective.**

Preliminary studies of two mRNA vaccines conducted with 30,000 to 40,000 patients each suggest that these vaccines may be greater than 90 percent effective. FDA review of these reports will likely confirm this, but it is unlikely that the vaccines will be this effective across the entire population once widely released in the community. Initial studies tend to exclude immune-compromised patients, and children and the very old, whose immune systems may respond differently to vaccination.

If a vaccine's true effectiveness is lower than reported in studies, but the population does not understand this, we may create a false sense of security. Or if people return to normal before we have reached the goal of widespread vaccination, interacting with others without following social distancing rules, we could see additional viral spread. In addition, once a vaccine is released, it is going to be challenging to convince patients who previously may have been interested in enrolling in a vaccine study to do so, and it is clear that to get to our goal of universal vaccination as quickly as possible we will need safe and effective vaccines from multiple pharmaceutical companies.

**3. The vaccine needs to be safe.**

Covid-19 is a deadly disease. The overwhelming majority of those who are infected by Covid-19 survive, but it still kills a tremendous number of people.

The mortality rate for a disease is measured using the following formula:

$$\text{Mortality Rate} = \frac{\text{Number of People Who Die of the Disease}}{\text{Number of People Infected with the Disease}}$$

In mid-April 2020, worldwide, there were approximately 140,000 Covid-19 deaths and two million people infected with the disease. This gave us a mortality rate of seven percent: 140,000 divided by 2,000,000, then multiplied by 100 to reach a percentage. By early October 2020, there were approximately one million deaths and over 38 million people infected worldwide, for a mortality rate of 2.6 percent. While lower than we had initially feared, this is still higher than the flu, which has a mortality rate between .01 and .02 percent and kills between 12,000 and 61,000 people a year in the U.S.

A virus's mortality rate changes when either the number of people who die of the disease (the numerator) or the number of people infected with the disease (the denominator) changes. With Covid-19, the mortality rate is dropping because of changes in both.

The numerator is now lower (relative to the denominator) because, increasingly, more people who contract Covid-19 survive the disease. There are two reasons for this. First, we have learned how to treat the disease more effectively. Second, the age of the average Covid-19 patient was much higher during the start of the pandemic than later on in the pandemic. Simply: more young people are getting infected now, and this population is less likely to die of the disease.

We have three theories to explain this change. First, young people may experience more exposure to the disease now than at the start of the pandemic (whether because they are less cautious, or because they are more likely to work in industries that do not allow them to work from home). Second, the use of aggressive safety measures for older, at-risk populations (such as nursing home residents) has lowered the infection rate among those groups. Lastly, Covid-19 may be mutating to become more infectious, and more so for young people.

At the same time, the denominator (the number of people infected with Covid-19) is expanding. We have learned that there are a lot of people who have the disease but are asymptomatic. As we expand testing, we identify more symptomatic and asymptomatic cases, which means that the number of recorded infections goes up.

These dynamics are pushing Covid-19's overall mortality rate lower.

A successful vaccine must produce benefits that far outweigh any risks and, like everything in medicine, there are risks to vaccines. In the case of polio, measles, and a host of other vaccines, the scales tilt strongly to the side of benefits. These vaccines cause little or no harm, and have nearly eradicated these diseases, saving millions of lives.

But that's not how it always works. Take the 1976 swine flu debacle, for example. The U.S. government was on high alert for the next pandemic and thought they had found it in the swine flu. Although the WHO recommended that the world "watch and wait" before determining if a vaccine was necessary, President Ford's administration aggressively pursued a campaign to vaccinate all Americans. Congress enacted a law that created the Swine Flu Immunization Program, and a vaccine – a variation of the flu shot – was rushed to market. In total, 45 million Americans were vaccinated.

In retrospect, most experts question the rationale of this vaccine program. There is a strong belief that it was politically motivated (Ford was in the midst of a presidential campaign and needed an issue around which to rally the country). The pandemic never developed, so the vaccine provided no benefit. But there were rare cases in which the vaccine recipients suffered long-lasting neurological damage.

I, along with most public health experts, believe that the benefits of an effective Covid-19 vaccine will be great. However, a vaccine given to hundreds of millions of people will likely have an adverse impact on some who receive the shot. As such, it is essential that the FDA not cut any corners and complete a full evaluation of every potential vaccine candidate.

Because we must we aim for universal vaccination, a vaccine with even a small adverse reaction rate (especially if that adverse reaction is a severe one) may have significant negative consequences for a segment of the population. FDA review and approval will help us evaluate this risk. I'm not a person who is opposed to vaccination – quite the contrary – but as with all medical treatments, we need to weigh risks against benefits in order to make an informed decision regarding a Covid-19 vaccine.

When I graduated medical school, I took the Hippocratic Oath. Most people – even most physicians – associate the phrase *Primum non nocere* with the Oath: "First do no harm." This phrase has always guided my practice of medicine. In my mind, it is the key component in assuring high-quality healthcare for our patients. We cannot completely remove the inherent risks that are part of medicine today, but we should strive to minimize those risks. Good science does that, but good science takes time. A rushed or bad vaccine could hurt, or even kill, people – but, to be clear, this is not the case with any FDA-approved vaccine, and I am optimistic that it will not be the case with vaccines hat the FDA thoroughly reviews.

**4. We would need to vaccinate billions of people all around the world.**

The world is becoming smaller and more connected. This is true of medicine, and very true of Covid-19. Covid-19 has moved around the world at a speed not seen before, overrunning hospitals and destroying economies around the globe. The expectation – and hope – is that the cure will spread around the world just as quickly.

This will be a major logistical challenge – producing billions of doses of the vaccine, producing billions of needles and syringes for administering the vaccine, and transporting these around a world with drastically reduced air capacity (most air freight of medical equipment is transported in the storage compartments of regular passenger flights), as well as reduced ocean shipping capacity. And some of the vaccines under development must be transported and stored at sub-freezing temperatures. This is never easy, but is especially difficult when dealing with such large quantities of a medication. Additionally, most vaccines under development require two doses separated by three to four weeks, doubling the number of doses, needles, and syringes required.

This raises issues of equity and priority – do "poor" countries have to wait until the "rich" countries complete their vaccinations to receive aid? More specifically, what happens to underprivileged people in poor countries? (I believe those in power in even the poorest of countries will have early access to an effective vaccine.)

And if the vaccine is expensive, who will cover the costs? This may be less of an issue in the U.S., where I expect that the government will pick up the costs related to the vaccine. But the cost of vaccinating other nations likely will be a significant portion of some countries' GDP. We have eradicated polio in the U.S., but we have not done so around the world. Why? Primarily because of the cost. We absolutely could eradicate it worldwide if wealthy countries made this a priority and provided the necessary resources and manpower to help other countries. For Covid-19, there has been talk of universal access to a vaccine, but we will have to wait and see what happens.

* * * * *

A typical vaccine consists of inactive live bacteria or virus (often grown in chicken or mammalian cells), or inactive proteins that have been removed from the surface of bacteria or viruses. These components are injected into patients to elicit an antibody response. If the patient later encounters that bacteria or virus, they are primed to produce antibodies and fight off the pathogen to prevent infection.

Many Covid-19 vaccines are not derived from samples of the virus itself, but rather from lab-synthesized Covid-19 mRNA (a molecule that makes proteins called "antigens"). When the vaccine is injected into the patient, the mRNA uses the patient's cellular infrastructure to produce Covid-19 antigens, which then trigger the body to produce Covid-19 antibodies, creating immunity. Scientists have investigated this mRNA technology both for cancer treatment and vaccine development. An mRNA vaccine has significant advantages: it is potentially safer because it does not require the use of chicken or other mammalian cells, it allows for rapid development and production of a vaccine, and it is relatively inexpensive compared to other methods of producing vaccines.

In theory, an mRNA vaccine is very safe. There is no use of actual bacteria or virus in its development, and the mRNA does not incorporate itself into the patient's DNA, as some people fear. Once the antigens are made, the body breaks down the mRNA. However, we do not have much experience with this technology. Preliminary results are encouraging, but no other vaccine that is available today uses this technology. It is difficult to be patient in the middle of a pandemic, but we must wait for the final results of clinical trials to determine these vaccines' effectiveness and safety.

Before I leave vaccines, let me be clear that I have very little patience for anti-vaxxers, people who oppose vaccinations. Anti-vaxxers choose to ignore science and spread baseless conspiracy theories. The original anti-vaxxer claim, that vaccines are linked to autism, has been repeatedly debunked. The study on which that claim is based has since been retracted, and the physician who ran it is now barred from practicing medicine in his home country, the United Kingdom.

Unfortunately, the anti-vaxxer movement has spread out of control, especially in the United States. Many anti-vaxxers claim that vaccines are always dangerous and cite a mistrust of harmful "chemicals" present in all vaccines. I think it is important to take a brief journey into these chemicals to specifically address these myths.

Thimerosal: Thimerosal is a preservative that prevents bacterial or fungal contamination. It is a form of mercury, but it is excreted from the body much more rapidly than the type of mercury found in fish, which can be harmful if consumed in large quantities. No scientific study has ever shown that thimerosal is linked to autism or has any other harmful effects. Because of pressure from the anti-vaccine movement, thimerosal has been removed from all vaccines with the exception of the annual flu shot, and there are thimerosal-free flu shots available.

Formaldehyde: Formaldehyde is used to inactivate viruses and detoxify bacterial toxins. It can cause cancer when consumed in large doses, but humans have small amounts of formaldehyde in our bodies that are part of our normal metabolism. The amount of formaldehyde in vaccines is negligible; the average newborn has 50-70 times more formaldehyde in their body than what is present in a single vaccine.

Aluminum: Aluminum is used as an adjuvant in vaccines to increase the body's immune response. This allows us to administer lower dosages and less frequent injections. Aluminum is naturally present in water, foods, and even breast milk. The amount of aluminum in a vaccine is so small that there is no discernible increase in aluminum levels after a vaccine is given. There is no scientific evidence that aluminum given in the small amounts present in a vaccine has any harmful effects.

Antibiotics: Antibiotics are used in the production process of vaccines to prevent bacterial contamination. They are almost completely removed during the final stages of vaccine purification. Even in patients with a known antibiotic allergy, the risk of a reaction from a vaccine is extremely low.

Gelatin: Gelatin is used as a preservative and stabilizer in vaccines. The chance of having an allergic reaction to gelatin is one in two million, and children with true gelatin allergies should receive an exemption for vaccines with gelatin.

Monosodium Glutamate (MSG): MSG is used as a preservative and stabilizer in adenovirus and influenza vaccines. A very small number of people may have a short-term reaction to MSG, but it is routinely used in numerous foods as a flavor enhancer. Decades of research have shown it to be safe.

Whether anti-vaxxers are unwilling to acknowledge the safety of these chemicals or are simply naive to the reality of the risk-benefit equation for vaccines, they needlessly put children and society at risk based on fake science, propaganda, and fear mongering. Aside from themselves and their children, they also selfishly put those who actually can't receive vaccines – like the immuno-compromised – at risk by lowering herd immunity.

Anti-vaxxing has serious, real-world consequences; from late 2014 to early 2015, the U.S. suffered a measles outbreak that infected over 100 people across seven states. This outbreak was linked to an infected person who had visited Disneyland, and the illness was spread by children whose parents had intentionally left them unvaccinated. If anti-vaxxers continue to refuse to vaccinate themselves and their children, we will see more outbreaks like this.

Anti-vaxxers expect zero risks from a vaccine, but many take actions with significantly greater risk every single day, like driving a car or playing a contact sport. They also ignore the tremendous benefits a vaccine can deliver.

We don't know the exact number of people who have avoided polio, mumps, measles, chickenpox, and, with the newer vaccines, cervical cancer, hepatitis, and meningitis, but the benefits in avoided death, improved quality of life, and avoided healthcare costs have been immeasurable.

When a safe and effective vaccine is available for Covid-19, the failure of a significant portion of the population to take it or the widespread belief that the vaccine is a silver bullet could prolong this pandemic unnecessarily. The virus could continue to spread or maybe even mutate to a more deadly strain. Alternatively, we could add Covid-19 to the list of diseases brought under control by an effective, safe, and widely-administered vaccine.

**The Real Numbers...**

- Vaccinations prevent an estimated 2-3 million deaths each year.
- The measles vaccine prevented 3.2 million deaths from 2000-2018.
- Every year, over 20 million children under the age of one do not receive vaccinations for diphtheria, pertussis, and tetanus, despite recommendations by the CDC and numerous other medical organizations.

CHAPTER TEN

# The Edison Approach

*"Never have I seen such a worldwide effort to tackle a disease head on – not to mention a new disease we know nothing about. We have made a lot of progress but there is still a long way to go."*

**Dr. Suraj Saggar**
Chief of Infectious Disease
Holy Name Medical Center

Most medical personnel, myself included, strive to practice evidence-based medicine. We treat patients based on what has been shown to be clinically effective. The alternative is the off-the-shelf approach – take something off the shelf that's not specifically intended to fix the problem and see if it works. I call this the Thomas Edison approach.

If you ever visit New Jersey, you should stop by the Edison National Historical Park and Laboratories in West Orange. There you will hear about the clock that supposedly stopped at the exact moment the great inventor died, and see the Black Maria, the studio where the first motion picture was filmed. (It was originally located on the Palisades, not too far from the Sisters of St. Joseph of Peace convent but has since been moved to the laboratories in West Orange.)

But what I find most intriguing at the Edison laboratories is the storage room. When I visited the museum as a child, an older man who worked for Edison retold the story of how Edison had struggled to find the right material to serve as the filament for his new invention, the lightbulb.

No matter what Edison used for the filament, after a few moments of giving off a glow, it burst into flames. He sent his agents out into the world to find alternatives – things that ended up on his shelf and that are now stored at the museum. The item I remember most is an elephant's ear, but the shelf was overflowing with a myriad of things from around the world.

In Edison's case, it turned out not to be the filament material which solved the problem, but the realization that if he removed the oxygen from the bulb, many filaments would glow rather than burn. But sometimes, the "off-the-shelf" approach works.

In medicine, there are times when good doctors will use the Edison approach to treat patients, rather than the evidence-based approach. When a patient is terminally ill, we often try – with the patient's permission – unproven treatments like new medicines or surgeries. Patients do not have much to risk at this stage, and this approach can sometimes lead to breakthroughs. The best-case scenario is that the patient improves and the timeline for the development of a treatment is shortened. The worst-case scenario is that the patient, who was already nearing death, dies sooner. But even then, we may uncover something about the new treatment that will help future patients.

But in general – whenever possible – I believe that we must continue to rely on evidence-based medicine for three reasons:

1. With diseases like Covid-19, most people get better with standard treatment, or even no treatment at all. If we try an off-the-shelf treatment, we may inaccurately attribute a patient's improvement to the treatment that has been administered when it was actually the result of the natural course of the virus.
2. Evidence-based medical studies don't just test for efficacy of a treatment, but also test to see what unexpected harm might occur.

3. Since we have limited resources, if we spend a great deal of time, effort, and money chasing off-the-shelf treatments, we may underinvest in the science that leads us to more mainstream treatments that, in the end, have the greatest potential for success.

I was once told of a rather clever scam. You write to 1,000 people and tell them you are clairvoyant and that you can successfully pick the winner of an upcoming football game between team A and team B. You tell 500 of those people that team A will win and tell the other 500 people that team B will win. You correctly predicted the winner for 500 people. You then send those 500 people predictions for another upcoming game, again telling half of them that one team will win and the other half that the other team will win. You do this for another week, and then tell the now-smaller group of 125, "I've been right three times in a row. I can tell you the name of next week's winning team, but this time, I need a check first." If all 125 people send you a check and place a big bet on that week's game, you'll make a tidy profit – and half of those 125 will win big. They'll be true believers, convinced that you were really clairvoyant.

Disease often works the same way. Not infrequently, patients who would have improved with no medical intervention are prescribed some form of treatment. When they get better, they attribute their improvement to the treatment they received.

One of my mentors during my residency, Dr. Robert Braham, told me that the most important thing to understand as a primary care physician is that 90 percent of patients will get better with no intervention (this might have been a bit of an exaggeration, but he was making a point). A good doctor spends most of their time treating the 10 percent who really need help, while trying to convince the patients who will get better on their own that they don't need any medical intervention – no medicine, no X-rays, no additional tests, no surgeries.

Throughout my career, Dr. Braham's advice has guided my practice of medicine.

I've always remembered his words of wisdom, and that is why I am extremely cautious about prescribing medications – all of which have potential side effects. Antibiotics are the best example of this.

In my early days of practice, patients frequently came in complaining of a runny nose or stuffed up sinuses. My most common response: "This is a viral infection, and you'll likely get better in three to five days." More often than not, the patients still requested antibiotics. I would explain, "Antibiotics have the potential for side effects and are not likely to help in this situation." Not infrequently, these conversations got a little contentious. But I would continue, "Look, I want to do what's best for you. I have a waiting room full of patients, and a wife and children waiting for me to come home. If I give you what you want, I can get home sooner. But what you want isn't what's best for you. Let me explain why...."

When I went on to explain the risks and benefits of antibiotics, that would do it for most people. Once they realized that I truly believed that antibiotics would not help and that I was committed to providing them the best possible care – care that, most of the time, did not require antibiotics – they would accept that their symptoms just needed to run their course without intervention.

Some patients, however, would leave my office (without antibiotics) and call a medical friend or family member to ask for a prescription (in Northern New Jersey, everyone seems to have a friend or relative who can write a prescription "in an emergency"). In some of these cases, the prescriptions given were for an even more powerful antibiotic than I would have prescribed, had I determined antibiotics were appropriate.

Many doctors tend to follow the path of least resistance when it comes to patient care. This has led to overprescribing medications and patients experiencing unnecessary side effects. It has become the norm in part because it takes so much time and energy to convince patients they don't need any treatment. This applies even to my own family members, who, like most patients, want a quick fix for whatever is ailing them. But as I do with my patients, I always take the time to tell my family that they likely do not need medical assistance (when I truly believe that to be the case).

Like all medications, antibiotics are not risk-free. Prescribing antibiotics may keep a patient happy, but there are three big downsides to their overuse:

1. Some people have allergic reactions to antibiotics, and these can be severe. While side effects to antibiotics vary based on the drug and person, they can include rashes, diarrhea, swelling of the face, and difficulty breathing.
2. Bacteria are becoming more resistant to antibiotics, and our discovery of new antibiotics is slowing. Micro-organisms are very good at mutating to survive. This includes mutating to avoid being destroyed by antibiotics. These mutated bacteria are called "superbugs," and they're incredibly difficult to treat.
3. There is a balance between "good" and "bad" bacteria in the gut. Antibiotics can kill off good bacteria and let bad bacteria, specifically *Clostridium Difficile*, flourish, causing colitis. This can lead to perforation of the intestine and even death in some patients. The risk of getting colitis increases every time a patient takes an antibiotic. It also increases with age.

When I realized how many patients went around me to obtain antibiotics, I changed the way I practiced. I still gave my anti-antibiotic spiel, but when I was not able to convince a patient, I wrote a prescription for the least powerful antibiotic available and told them not to fill it for at least three days to see if they improved on their own. This strategy was an attempt to prevent patients from receiving (and using) a more powerful antibiotic from another physician. Most patients felt better with that piece of paper in hand, knowing they could fill it if they didn't improve on their own. In fact, most never did fill it. But others went straight to their pharmacy, took the antibiotic right away, and also got better (most would have anyway).

How does all of this apply to Covid-19? Let's turn for a moment to hydroxychloroquine.

Hydroxychloroquine is a drug that is traditionally used to fight malaria and lupus. During the early stages of the pandemic, there were patients, doctors, and politicians, including President Trump, who were convinced that hydroxychloroquine was effective in treating Covid-19. It was widely prescribed, and many patients got better. However, most patients with Covid-19 do get better, even without treatment.

So, the question is, what was the impact of the drug? The best studies show that hydroxychloroquine has no positive impact when tested against a placebo. Some hydroxychloroquine studies were actually stopped early because they showed that the drug caused an increase in cardiac deaths. Continuing those studies would have unethically put people in harm's way.

Hydroxychloroquine's risk of heart complications is actually well known due to its use in malaria and lupus patients. But the use of hydroxychloroquine to treat these diseases is acceptable because the known benefits outweigh the known risks. With Covid-19, there is still no evidence that hydroxychloroquine provides any benefits – though it still has its believers among recovered patients and their physicians. Mike took hydroxychloroquine when he contracted Covid-19 and ultimately had a strong recovery. He is confident this was because of the drug.

Without new data from studies, I remain skeptical.

It is possible that hydroxychloroquine may have a positive impact on patients depending on their stage of infection or when prescribed in a different dosage than those studied. However, absent any studies that prove it is effective, I do not believe that hydroxychloroquine should be prescribed to treat Covid-19. We should instead spend our time and efforts on drugs that have a better chance for success.

Our treatment of Covid-19 has consisted of steady but painstakingly slow steps forward. Early in the pandemic, Suraj and I brainstormed what "cocktail" of antiviral drugs might effectively fight the disease. (We call them cocktails, but they're actually a group of medications, or even just one pill that includes several drugs.) With no other options and too many very sick patients, we resorted to the off-the-shelf Edison approach. We created a cocktail for a handful of patients based on our educated guesses of what might work. Not unexpectedly, we saw no clear-cut improvements to their health.

Throughout the next few weeks and months, the medical community tried a variety of drugs to treat Covid-19, some effective and some not. At Holy Name, we learned a lot, and we made some small but real advancements with treatments that have since been confirmed to be effective by evidence-based, controlled scientific studies.

**On June 20, 2020**

- Six Trump campaign staff test positive prior to a rally in Tulsa.
- One thousand people test positive at a German meat plant.
- An outdoor movie theater opens at Miami's Hard Rock Stadium.

CHAPTER ELEVEN

# Treatments: Slow and Steady

*"There was a sense of despair at first.*
*Nothing seemed to help and patient after patient was dying.*
*Gradually we saw progress, but slower than many of us had hoped."*

**Arlene Van Dyk**
Critical Care RN
Holy Name Medical Center

A few weeks into the pandemic, as our medical and nursing staffs worked tirelessly, frustration was growing. Despite the staff's best efforts, many people were dying, and we had no effective treatments.

Feelings of frustration are all too common amongst healthcare professionals, even when there is not a pandemic. The harsh reality is that we still are not very good at treating, let alone curing, many diseases – pancreatic cancer, ALS (Lou Gehrig's Disease), and Alzheimer's disease all have no known cure and few treatments. With Covid-19, our frustration at a lack of effective treatments was exacerbated by the sudden and enormous volume of patients, our complete lack of knowledge about how this new disease affects the body, and its deadly impact on previously healthy people. To be honest, we felt completely helpless.

There was a palpable sense of relief when some drugs finally began to show promise.

**Remdesivir: A drug that decreases viral replication. It was initially used to**

**treat Ebola, but was not found to be effective against it.**

We received permission to use remdesivir to treat Covid-19 patients through the FDA's expanded access (EA) program, also called the "compassionate use" program. The EA program gives certain patients access to "investigational medical products" that would not ordinarily be available. To be eligible for treatment under the EA program, a patient needed to have all three of the following:

- A serious or immediate life-threatening disease or condition.
- No comparable or satisfactory alternative therapy.
- Potential benefits that justify the potential risks of the treatment.

Getting permission for use of remdesivir was not easy. Dr. Ravit Barkama, who oversees our clinical research department, spent hours on the phone and sending emails to the FDA and Gilead (the manufacturer of remdesivir), giving details on each patient we thought could benefit. Interestingly, Ravit learned that both the FDA and Gilead were more likely to approve a patient if she called late at night. She hypothesized that the employees who worked these "off" hours had more authority to independently approve applications. Initially, we received permission to intravenously administer remdesivir to six critically ill patients. We had minimal hope for their recovery, but remarkably, two of them survived. This was a better outcome than we had expected, but six patients was certainly not a large enough sample to draw any conclusions.

As the FDA and Gilead started approving our applications, our relief that there was a potential new treatment was tempered by a new frustration: there wasn't much remdesivir available. Under EA regulations, which patients could receive remdesivir, when they could get it, and how much they could be given was completely controlled by the FDA and Gilead.

About a week after we began administering remdesivir to these six patients, I ran into Ravit in the hall. She appeared harried, and as soon as she saw me, she blurted out, "I need to have a difficult conversation with you." There was no one else within earshot, so we talked quietly in the hallway.

"We have an issue," she said. "One of our remdesivir patients just died and we have leftover medication. We're supposed to return it to Gilead, but we have several other patients who I think could benefit from it. Is there any way we can give it to them?"

This was a really tough ethical question. We were in the midst of a pandemic that was killing so many of our patients, and there was a chance that this medicine could save lives. However, the rules were clear: we could not give this medicine to any patients without approval from both the FDA and the manufacturer.

But I wanted to make sure that I fully understood the situation. Was there any way around this? What were the implications of breaking this rule? Might we be barred from future studies? We debated and discussed and, sadly, we both agreed that we could not give the leftover medication to unapproved patients.

The medicine was in short supply and should be returned so that approved patients at other facilities could potentially benefit from it. It was a deeply dissatisfying decision, but breaking the rules would have had serious consequences, both for the hospital and for individual patients.

Several days later, I again ran into Ravit in the hallway. I asked her if she had already returned the remdesivir. She told me she had not and, for a brief second, I was concerned that she had disregarded our conversation. That was not the case, she explained. Instead, she had decided to contact Gilead and explain the situation. After several calls, she ultimately received permission from Gilead to give the leftover medicine to another patient.

When more remdesivir became available, we treated well over 100 patients who met the FDA's criteria. On June 1, 2020, Gilead put out a press release announcing that remdesivir, when given early, did not reduce mortality in Covid-19 patients, but did reduce the length of hospital stays. The formal study was fully released in October. This brought us all a glimmer of hope; based on our experience, we thought additional research might show that changing the dose or timing of administration might have an even greater effect. After this study, Gilead made even more remdesivir available, and we were able to secure doses for another 80 patients. We finally reached a point where remdesivir was given to any Covid-19 patient who had decreased oxygen levels and was sick enough to be admitted to the hospital.

Like the treatment for HIV/AIDS, we may find in time that the ultimate treatment for Covid-19 is a cocktail of drugs, of which remdesivir will only be a part. It is difficult to know. What is clear however, is that remdesivir is not a miracle drug. Used by itself, its overall benefit is real, but small.

**Steroids: Powerful anti-inflammatories with mixed reports of success and failure for the treatment of Covid-19.**

Steroids are often used to treat inflammation in the body (e.g., a bad case of poison ivy or an acute attack of arthritis). They can also have a positive impact on certain critically ill patients – but not without some negative side effects. Inflammation is essential in fighting infections, and steroids can suppress this inflammation, making the infection even worse.

For some patients, however, the inflammation caused by infections becomes a problem in and of itself. Specifically, too much inflammation in the lungs can cause acute respiratory distress syndrome (ARDS). The inflammation overwhelms the lungs, fills the lungs with fluid, and prevents the essential transfer of oxygen from the air the patient breathes to the patient's blood. On the X-ray of a healthy patient, the lungs are clearly visible. On an X-ray of someone with severe ARDS, the lungs can completely be "whited out" – it actually looks like someone took a paintbrush and painted over the lungs with white paint.

There was a consensus among our critical care and infectious disease physicians that treatment with remdesivir made sense during the early infectious stage of Covid-19 and that treatment with steroids made sense during the later inflammatory stage. But these were educated guesses.

In July, a study was released that confirmed those guesses. When compared to a control group, Covid-19 patients who received dexamethasone (a specific steroid) had reduced mortality.

**Actemra: An interleukin-6 blocking agent that also has powerful anti-inflammatory effects and is used to treat rheumatoid arthritis and certain cancers.**

Dr. Thomas Birch, our Director of Infection Control, sought me out after reading a small study of 21 patients from China. The study suggested that Actemra might be helpful in counteracting inflammation in Covid-19 patients.

We agreed to use Actemra "off label" (in a way not yet proven or suggested by the manufacturer, but allowed under FDA rules) and ultimately gave it to more than 245 patients, spending over $1 million on the drug. We believe that Actemra had a powerful impact on our patients. We administered it to three members of the Holy Name medical staff who were quite ill with Covid-19. Their response was astounding – their fevers decreased, their oxygen levels improved, and they stayed off ventilators. We did not know for sure whether their dramatic clinical changes were caused by the Actemra, but the timing and the pattern were hard to ignore.

While we feel strongly that Actemra has a significant clinical benefit, preliminary studies have shown mixed results. We are anxiously awaiting the results of more definitive studies and are hopeful that they will confirm our suspicion that Actemra can help treat Covid-19.

**Placental Stem Cells: Cells harvested from placentas. These cells have been used for treatment of certain cancers and genetic disorders.**

For several years, Holy Name, in partnership with Pluristem, an Israeli pharmaceutical company, has been investigating the use of placental stem cells for leg re-vascularization (in which the blood vessels in a patient's leg are opened up).

This re-vascularization can be done using intravascular balloons or by surgical intervention, but there are clinical situations in which these two options are not viable. Pluristem, with our assistance, is testing whether placental stem cell injections might be a useful third option. In certain situations, the body can re-vascularize on its own. The heart and legs can develop collateral circulation – additional blood flow that circumvents blockages – and placental stem cells may assist this process.

In Israel, Pluristem had used these placental stem cells in the treatment of Covid-19 with some success and was looking for a U.S. partner to further study this treatment. Ravit had a relationship with Pluristem so Holy Name was a natural fit. With the FDA's consent, we were permitted to use this treatment for select Covid-19 patients through the EA program.

We administered stem cells to four critically ill patients, and all four survived. One was Edward Pierce, the Associate Scenic Designer for the Broadway musical *Wicked* (who also has worked on more than 20 other Broadway shows). He has since appeared on national television to talk about his experience with Covid-19, the use of stem cells, and how the disease changed his life. When he left the hospital after three weeks on a ventilator, we played "Defying Gravity" from *Wicked* over the loudspeakers.

Holy Name was the first hospital in the U.S. to pioneer placental stem cells on Covid-19 patients. Our efforts have contributed to the launch of a more formal study.

**Plasma Therapy: A treatment in which the plasma (the liquid part of blood) of a patient who has survived Covid-19 is injected into another patient battling the virus.**

In April 2020, a very small study in China suggested that plasma therapy might be beneficial to Covid-19 patients. If previously infected patients now have Covid-19 antibodies in their plasma that helped them recover from the disease, the thought is that these antibodies could help other patients when introduced to their systems.

Plasma infusions have successfully been used to treat diphtheria, polio, rabies, and, more recently, Ebola. Despite these successes, we generally try to avoid plasma treatment because it comes from human blood which, although relatively safe, poses some inherent risks.

Early in the pandemic, there was an inadequate supply of plasma, which had to be donated by patients who had survived Covid-19. But once it became available, we did use it with the FDA's permission. Initial results of plasma treatment for Covid-19 are encouraging. However, the treatment is still under evaluation and we await the results of larger, well-designed studies.

**Monoclonal Antibodies: Medications that are synthesized in a laboratory and mimic the antibodies that the human body produces.**

Toward the end of our first surge of patients, we entered into a study with Regeneron, a Tarrytown, New York-based pharmaceutical company, on the use of monoclonal antibodies in Covid-19 patients. You may recall that the Covid-19 virus has spikes on its surface. Regeneron created a cocktail of monoclonal antibodies targeted specifically at these spikes.

This study has three arms:

1. Prophylaxis (prevention) for patients who have had significant household exposure to a known Covid-19 patient but have so far tested negative.
2. Treatment of Covid-19 patients who do not require hospitalization.
3. Treatment of Covid-19 patients who do require hospitalization.

In these double-blinded studies, two out of three patients received treatment with the anti-spike protein and one out of three received a placebo. Holy Name was the first hospital in the world to treat a patient with this experimental treatment.

When President Trump was hospitalized with Covid-19 in October 2020, he received this medication – not as part of a study, but through the FDA emergency use authorization program. In November, the FDA expanded access to treatment to all qualifying patients though the EA program.

The treatment is a one-time infusion, and while the study is not complete, initial results suggest that patients have decreased symptoms and no significant side effects. But as discussed, good science takes time, and we need to wait for the completion of these studies to truly evaluate this medication's efficacy.

**Good Old-Fashioned Nursing**

Sometimes the best treatments come not from a drug or fancy equipment, but simply from good nursing. For example, a major challenge with Covid-19 is its impact on the lungs. Lungs infected with Covid-19 do not adequately transport oxygen to the blood, so to assist with oxygen flow, we used a technique called proning.

Proning is simply positioning a patient on their belly. It helps a patient use parts of the lungs that typically are not utilized, resulting in increased oxygen flow from the lungs to the blood. Proning is used to treat a variety of illnesses that affect a patient's ability to breathe, such as certain types of severe pneumonia. For Covid-19, we modified this process a bit when our nurses realized that rotating a patient not just onto their belly but also onto their left and right sides improved blood oxygen levels. The Covid-19 ward at Holy Name was full of patients on their sides, on their backs, or on their stomachs, however we could position them to help them use their entire lungs, keep their blood oxygenated, and keep them off a ventilator.

For those patients who did need a ventilator, flipping them onto their stomach for 15 minutes every hour helped considerably improve blood oxygen levels. This was a difficult process for these patients, who were attached to several IV tubes and a ventilator. It required six to eight staff members, all attired in PPE, to accomplish the maneuver. Our nursing team coordinated these movements, and we developed a team approach reliant on staff whose main focus was proning patients.

I would be remiss not to mention ventilators again. Hospitals and healthcare workers learning how to better utilize ventilators for Covid-19 patients has definitely contributed to lowering the Covid-19 mortality rate. First, the realization that patients did better when kept off ventilators as long as possible was a true breakthrough. Second, as the pandemic progressed, our staff developed a better understanding of how to balance the need for oxygen with the desire to not put undue pressure on the lungs. Determining the proper ventilator adjustments for each patient in each situation is as much art as it is science, and we collectively improved as we learned from our patients.

* * * * *

There's an old saying: "The doctor who treats himself has a fool for a patient." I'm not a fool (at least not as far as medical treatment), but I do know what I would do and how I would like to be treated were I to get sick with Covid-19. With the data and experience we have today, this is how I would want to be treated:

1. After initial diagnosis with a swab, I would go on strict home quarantine (assuming I did not need hospitalization) for at least two weeks, longer if my symptoms persisted (home quarantine needs to extend three days after the last symptoms or a minimum of two weeks, whichever is longer). I would attempt to enroll in the Regeneron monoclonal antibody study and hopefully receive the one-time infusion.

2. During my home quarantine, I would treat my symptoms: increase fluids, take acetaminophen or ibuprofen, and rest. I would not take hydroxychloroquine.

3. If I began to feel short of breath while resting, I would be admitted to Holy Name with careful oxygen monitoring, and oxygen administration. I would want to start remdesivir and steroids. If I had not been able to enroll in the Regneron study, I would attempt to access monoclonal antibody treatment through the FDA's EA program.

4. If my symptoms progressed and my oxygen levels decreased, I would add Actemra, high-flow oxygen, and proning to my treatment.

5. If, despite these interventions, I continued to worsen, I would request plasma treatment.

6. I would tell the doctors that they should hold off on ventilator support for as long as possible, understanding that this does create some increased

risk of waiting too long and could increase my risk for other problems, including strokes or even death.

7. If, despite all of these measures, I required intubation and ventilator support, I would have the doctors add placental stem cells. Eileen, who is my healthcare proxy, would be in close contact with the medical team for regular updates. Based on their assessment of the situation, I would expect her, in accordance with my advanced directive, to approve continued aggressive care until they felt that further treatment was futile.
8. At that point, I would want Eileen to take me off the ventilator and allow me to die as peacefully as possible. In other circumstances, I would want her and our children at my side, but if I were sick with Covid-19, this would likely be unsafe for them.

I lay out these eight steps of Covid-19 treatment in an attempt to educate the reader as to where we stand with existing treatments. The treatments will change and evolve as we learn more through additional studies and experience. If you contract Covid-19, please immediately quarantine, then consult your doctor to establish a course of treatment if necessary.

The vast majority of patients will never get past step two above. But a small percentage of patients and their families will unfortunately face more progressive symptoms, and an even smaller percentage will reach the eighth step. Today, this is the sad reality of Covid-19.

**On July 10, 2020**

- The United Kingdom eases Covid-19 travel restrictions for a dozen countries – but not the U.S.
- California releases 8,000 prisoners early following a Covid-19 outbreak at the facility.
- Georgia reactivates a makeshift hospital at Atlanta's convention center.
- A New York gym owner sues the state over not being able to re-open.

CHAPTER TWELVE

# Yes, Death Gets Its Own Chapter

*"Death is not the opposite of life, but a part of it."*

**Haruki Murakami**
Author

Victoria was admitted to the hospital with typical Covid-19 symptoms. She was HIV-positive and had lived with HIV/AIDS for more than 10 years. She had beaten breast cancer. She was a single mom who, through all her hardships, had raised a son, Dante, who had become a successful lawyer. Victoria worsened after a few days in the hospital and was transferred to the ICU, where she was placed on a ventilator. Ten days later, she became our first patient to successfully be taken off a ventilator. The ICU was ecstatic – successes were rare at the time – and Dante breathed a sigh of relief. We all knew what Victoria had gone through and were thrilled that she had beaten Covid-19.

After she came off the ventilator, Victoria informed her care team that if she were to suffer a setback, she did not want to be put back on it. An order was placed making her a "do not resuscitate" (DNR).

Dante, who lived in the Midwest and was unable to be physically present for his mother's illness, was distraught at her decision. He pleaded with her to change her mind. He also requested that the care team not accept the DNR order. The discussion became contentious, so I referred it to our ethics committee.

From an ethical and legal perspective, it was a fairly straightforward case. Victoria had full capacity to make this decision and we were ethically and legally obligated to support it. Dante struggled to understand. He could not accept that Victoria, who had fought all her life, was now ready to die if she could not recover without aggressive measures.

Our palliative team facilitated a conversation via iPad for the mother and son. The conversation, as expected, was incredibly emotional, but eventually Dante agreed that his mom's wishes should be respected. If she were to worsen and develop "air hunger" (the common term for the discomfort a patient feels when they are severely short of breath), instead of being placed back on a ventilator, Victoria would be given morphine intravenously to relieve her discomfort.

We hoped and expected that Victoria would recover and that the plan she had put in place would not be needed. Unfortunately, within a couple of days, her breathing again became labored. As she worsened, she was placed on a continuous drip of intravenous morphine and died, comfortably, within 12 hours.

I felt the unfairness of a woman who had held off HIV/AIDS, beaten back cancer, and successfully raised a son on her own, but was killed by what some were still describing as "just a bad flu."

* * * * *

I have mixed feelings about including a chapter on death. American culture dictates that we don't talk about death. Many people, when talking about someone in their own life who has died, will use the term "passed" instead, especially when talking to children.

I think, as a society, we need to be more open about death, more contemplative about how we want to die, and more deliberate in controlling the circumstances of our death. So, death has its own chapter. It's going to happen to us all, so we may as well face it head on.

The first time I remember encountering death, I was eight years old. I was very fond of our neighbor, Mr. Darrow. He was one of two brothers who each owned a house across the street from ours. His children were about 10 years older than my siblings and me, and the rest of the neighborhood kids looked up to them. The Darrows always welcomed kids of all ages into their home or to play in their yard – usually a game of "kick the can."

I have a vivid memory of learning about Mr. Darrow's sudden death from my mother. When she told me, I ran to my room, lay on my bed, curled up into a ball, and sobbed. After a few minutes, my mother came into my room and, very compassionately, but also very matter-of-factly, talked to me about the reality of death. It was okay to be sad, she said, but I needed to understand that death was a part of life. We needed to hold those who died in our memory, even as we moved on. She told me to take whatever time I needed, and then to come out of my room and join the rest of the family for dinner.

This conversation with my mother and her approach to the reality of death set the tone for my future experiences with ill and dying patients. Throughout my career, I have seen a lot of dead bodies. I speak frankly about death with patients, family, friends, and colleagues.

Patients' families have told me that I communicate the reality of their loved one's illness and death in an easy-to-understand, factual way. This is not out of a lack of compassion; in fact, it is the opposite. Death is a reality we are all going to face and, in facing it squarely, we can lessen the heartache that accompanies it.

This is also how I approach the death of my own loved ones.

There is a beautiful, tranquil place tucked away on the banks of the Saddle River, the Villa Marie Claire, located about 15 minutes from Holy Name. For decades, it was a retreat for the Sisters of St. Joseph of Peace. In 2010, the sisters donated the Villa to Holy Name on the condition that it become a permanent hospice center.

Patients go to the Villa to die. But not in the way most Americans die, hooked up to medical equipment in a desperate effort to extend life a day, an hour, or a minute. Patients at the Villa die in a deliberate, peaceful fashion. They plan ahead and die on their own terms.

The Villa is staffed by an interdisciplinary team of professionals, all of whom are trained in interfaith and multicultural traditions. The staff structures care for the medical, emotional, and spiritual needs of a patient nearing their end of life. And it is important to note that while hospice is mostly about caring for the patient, it also is about caring for the patient's family or loved ones by providing for their emotional needs.

My father died at the Villa Marie Claire surrounded by his children, and his experience further motivated me to be an advocate for planning a peaceful death. That is how I want to die.

Eileen's father also died at the Villa, the day after his 85th birthday. The day prior to his death, his wife and their eight children, with assorted spouses and grandchildren in tow, gathered around him and sang "Take Me Out to the Ball Game." I remember thinking that the song was a great choice for my former baseball coach – he was a devoted Yankees fan. When the group reached the line "One, two, three strikes you're out," Eileen and I exchanged a look; the lyric had a different meaning when sung at the deathbed of a man who had beaten two cancers and was now succumbing to a third. But when the family looks back at his death now, I have to admit that we laugh about that song.

Unlike my father and Eileen's father, Covid-19 patients did not have the option to choose how they wanted to die. Dying of Covid-19 was an isolating experience, and it was very clear that patients, families, and staff were going to face death in a way that was previously unimaginable. The harsh reality is that Covid-19 patients die without the presence or support of the ones they love.

To protect family members and the community at large, Holy Name, like other hospitals, did not allow any visitation in the midst of the pandemic. The administrative team grappled long and hard as we tried to develop an alternative. Could we allow visitors to wear PPE? Could we limit visitation instead of banning it completely? Ultimately, the decision was made for us as Governor Murphy signed an executive order that completely banned hospital visitation. This must not have been an easy decision for him; however, I do believe it was the right decision and that it decreased the spread of Covid-19.

The ban on visitation contributed to Holy Name's eerie atmosphere. The hospital did not look or feel like a war zone, as one reporter stated, but more like something out of a futuristic dystopian novel. Non-clinical staff worked from home, there was no visitor foot traffic in the hallways, and we strongly felt the absence of chaplains, medical students, therapy dogs (and their owners), and our regular volunteers.

The quiet halls were frequently interrupted by the scramble to reach a patient in cardiac arrest. Unfortunately, death was an all too frequent visitor on the wards.

Since family members were not allowed at the hospital, we made extra efforts to keep communication flowing between patients and their families. Our nurses did their best using FaceTime, Skype, Zoom, and Google Meet to keep patients in touch with their loved ones. Having some form of communication was unbelievably valuable to the patients and their families, but it in no way replaced the in-person interactions that they would have had under normal circumstances. Having loved ones nearby can be a pleasant distraction for sick patients, but more importantly, it is an essential component of both a healthy recovery and the dying process. Being with family and friends is good for the soul; virtual communication does not have the same impact for either patients or visitors.

Under normal circumstances, a critical care physician keeps an ICU patient's family informed of their loved one's status and, if necessary, informs the family if the patient has died. In the age of Covid-19, our critical care physicians were overwhelmed with direct patient care. They simply didn't have time to also manage communications with families. I decided that we needed to shift the responsibility of communicating with families about all issues, including end-of-life issues, away from these doctors.

Instead, we created a team of physicians, many of whom were available because elective procedures and surgeries had stopped, whose main function became communicating with families. Before talking with a patient's family, a member of this team reviewed the patient's medical records and had a brief discussion with the treating physician. These conversations with families focused on the patient's condition, treatment options (including experimental treatments), and, when necessary, end-of-life care.

When possible, we tried to assign each patient a single physician so that the family had one point of contact and knew who to speak with to get information. We aimed to build trust and consistency that families could rely on throughout a patient's stay at the hospital.

Often, one of the key areas of discussion was how to balance a patient's pain and alertness. Toward the end of life, patients often require large doses of medication to be kept comfortable. These medications sedate the patient and reduce their alertness. This balancing act becomes much easier if the patient or their family have made their wishes known. I have had patients who were adamant that they wanted to be aware and alert, no matter the pain, until the end. Others wanted no pain, even if it meant they were not able to interact with those around them.

This difficult decision is even harder on families and patients when they have not discussed the subject prior to an illness. Family members often disagree with each other or the patient. These types of discussions are always challenging, but they are considerably harder when conducted virtually.

Discussing a worsening prognosis or possible withdrawal of care with a patient's family was an even tougher conversation. Most times, the family wanted to see their loved one, one last time. The electronic communication facilitated by the nurses additionally provided some level of assurance that the medical team was pursuing an appropriate course of action.

However, the inability to be physically present with dying loved ones will likely have long-term psycho-social impacts on patients' family members.

* * * * *

We had heard of hospitals in Europe that, when faced with a shortage of ventilators, had had to decide which patients would be put on the machines and which would not, a literal life or death decision. As the number of Covid-19 patients grew at Holy Name, we were concerned we might face the same difficult decisions.

Holy Name has always had an active ethics committee, which reviews cases that involve tough ethical choices. The ethics committee's role is not to make these decisions, but to provide guidance to patients, families, and the care team to help them make the decisions. The committee is made up of clinicians, legal counsel, nuns, administrators, and members of the Teaneck community. Over the years, the ethics committee has dealt with end-of-life issues, issues related to healthcare proxies, the occasional times when we have had to weigh risk between patients (a mother and her unborn child during a particularly risky delivery, for instance), or, as with Victoria and Dante, when patients' children do not agree with their parents' end-of-life choices.

At the start of the pandemic, I asked the ethics committee to evaluate a system for prioritizing care for those most in need. I wanted to have procedures in place before a crisis arose.

Working with the ethics committee, our palliative care team developed a tool to measure severity of illness for critically ill Covid-19 patients. This system considered factors such as age, comorbidities, and degree of lung dysfunction. If we faced a ventilator shortage, we decided, we would use these factors to determine which patients would be placed on the machines – namely, those with the best chance of surviving with the ventilator's help. The alternative would have been a first-come, first-served model; the ethics committee felt that that would be inappropriate and agreed that the patient scoring tool was the best approach.

At least once a day, we "scored" and "ranked" each critically ill Covid-19 patient so that we would be ready if we had to ration resources. We always knew which patients were the most likely to benefit from the treatment, and therefore who would receive it if we did not have enough ventilators for every patient. If we faced the unthinkable, we were prepared. Though we came within hours of having to use this ranking system, we fortunately never did.

* * * * *

Footage of large, refrigerated trucks that had been converted to morgues in New York City made the national news. So many people were dying in New York City that there was nowhere else to put the bodies. I was aghast when, three weeks into the crisis on one of our daily calls, I heard the CMO of another Northern New Jersey hospital mention that they needed to bring in a refrigerated truck because their morgue was full. Within the week, Holy Name needed one as well.

Before Covid-19, in a typical month at Holy Name, we had 5 to 10 deaths. In the first three months of Covid-19, we had 251.

Ordinarily, when someone dies at Holy Name, their body is transported to a local funeral home shortly after, usually within hours. But I had not anticipated that, like hospitals, funeral homes would be overrun by Covid-19. At the peak of the crisis, funeral homes were unable to accept bodies for days.

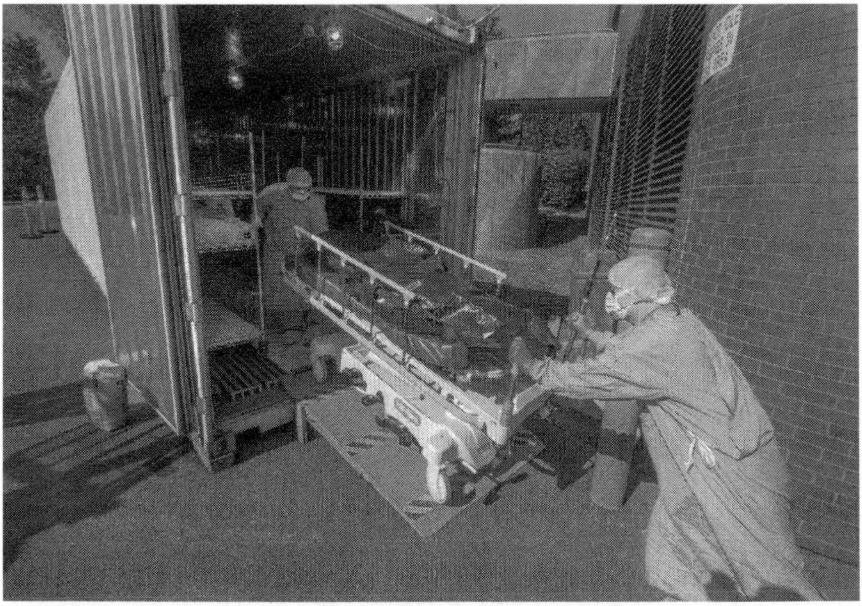

Using refrigerated trucks as morgues was an unfortunate necessity during the first wave of Covid-19 for many hospitals.

Since so many more patients were dying and funeral homes could not take them immediately, we created a special dedicated team of staff to prepare and transport bodies to the morgue or, if necessary, to the temporary refrigerated truck morgue. We even developed an enhanced logging system to track the deceased so that when funeral homes were able to come for pick up, we easily could locate the right body.

Of course, we always treat human remains with dignity – not just out of respect for the person who has died, but also out of respect for their family. During Covid-19, this became harder due to the sheer number of deaths, the fear of infection, and government regulations.

Something you don't see on medical shows is that dead bodies can be messy – they leak fluids. This is particularly true of patients who die after a long critical care hospitalization. To keep staff safe, Don found specially reinforced, heavy-duty remains bags. We didn't know for sure at the time whether dead bodies could transmit Covid-19 – and neither did the CDC or the WHO. During the first Covid-19 wave, both the CDC and the WHO issued guidance on the handling of the deceased. Not only did these two sets of guidelines conflict with each other, but they were based on experience with other infections, not Covid-19.

We wanted to do everything possible to protect our staff, and thus treated the remains of our Covid-19 patients as if they were infectious.

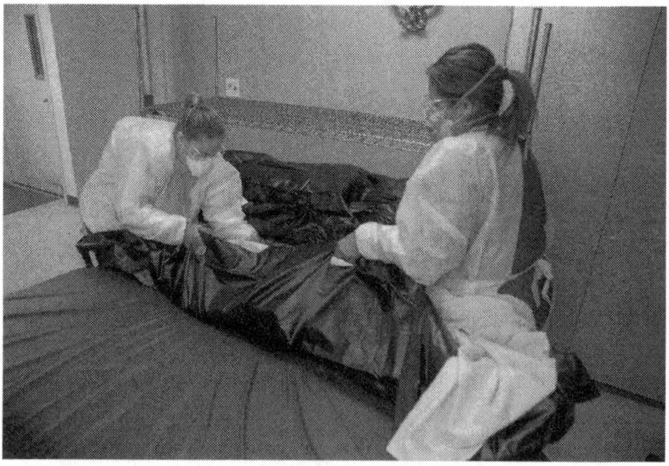

Covid-19 necessitated the use of heavy-duty body bags.

Because families were not allowed in the hospital at the time, it was necessary for a loved one to identify the deceased before the body was placed in a casket or crematorium. Funeral directors, who were instructed by the New Jersey Department of Health to interact with the bodies as little as possible, would unzip the body bag, take a photo, and send it to the family for identification. These photos were tough on the families in the best circumstances. To make things worse, there were times when the body's eyes and mouth, which the nurses at the hospital had closed, had opened during transport to the funeral home. The funeral directors had been told not to touch the bodies, so sometimes the eyes and mouth were open in the photos.

Both the CDC and the WHO have since updated their guidance. As of July 2020, the CDC has stated that it is unlikely that a dead body will transmit Covid-19. More specifically, under current CDC guidelines, families can even be involved in the preparation of the body with appropriate precautions, including PPE, and can have viewings with limited numbers of mourners following appropriate social distancing rules.

I think most people at some time in their lives (perhaps a number of times) wonder what happens to a dead body. In 2004, when a colleague of mine recommended a book about this subject, I was intrigued. *Stiff: The Curious Lives of Human Cadavers*, by Mary Roach, was a *New York Times* bestseller.

The book is a factual, fascinating, and, at times, explicit and humorous look at what happens to the human body after death. I couldn't put the book down and strongly recommend it for anyone who wants to put death in perspective – with a caveat. Some may find the book too explicit about the reality of what happens to our bodies.

* * * * *

During normal operations, an in-house physician pronounces patients dead. During the pandemic, we needed to modify this process. Most nurses are not allowed to pronounce a patient dead, but hospice nurses can, so we drew on them to take over this responsibility. Our hospice nurses also proved invaluable as they attempted to connect patients and their families one last time before death. Then after death, the hospice nurses prepared the body. They removed any tubes or IV lines, washed the body, and wrapped it in white sheets. This small change in our process relieved the primary nurses of much of these time-consuming and emotionally draining tasks, allowed them to concentrate their efforts on their other patients, and gave the hospice nurses the chance to provide another level of compassionate communication with loved ones.

While discussing end-of-life care can be an upsetting experience, we all should think about what kind of care we want to receive in our final days. It is key to record our wishes in advance directives – documents that provide instructions regarding healthcare wishes when we are no longer able to give those instructions ourselves. A well-crafted advance directive always improves the quality of care that patients receive and, just as importantly, assures that your wishes are carried out when you can no longer make healthcare decisions for yourself.

The majority of patients who do not have advance directives go on ventilators in the last stages before death. Going on a ventilator prolongs life, but in my mind, in many cases, it simply prolongs the act of dying, and does so with great discomfort and low quality of life.

Those thinking of putting a loved one on a ventilator near the end of life need to understand that it is a harrowing, miserable experience. My family knows that when I am dying, I do not want to be placed on a ventilator. When healthcare providers discuss this topic among themselves, the majority feel the same way. And many patients do as well. Victoria certainly did.

**Why are so many people still dying in the hospital?** ("Where People Die" by Dr. Robert H. Shmerling, Harvard Health Blog, October 31, 2018)

- A hope that medical care can cure the incurable.
- Lack of alternatives.
- The culture of medicine still focuses on cure and treatment instead of palliation.
- A healthcare reimbursement system that focuses on short-term in-patient care instead of long-term home care.

CHAPTER THIRTEEN

# Sorry Randi, No Easy Answers

*"On the [Covid-19] testing issue, this is one of our darkest moments in public health. I can't remember a time we've failed to do what we should have done. When South Korea can test more people in one day than we've been able to test in eight weeks, that should tell you we have a problem."*

**Dr. Michael T. Osterholm**
Director, Center for Infectious Disease Research and Policy
University of Minnesota
April 17, 2020

It had been a long day at the hospital, and I was doing my best to socially distance from Eileen – hard to do in a one-bedroom, 850-square-foot Manhattan apartment, but we were trying. I was lounging on the sofa, now also my temporary bed, when I received a call from my sister, Randi, who is a nurse for a home health agency in Connecticut.

"Adam, I was exposed to Covid-19 at work. Josh" – her husband – "is really nervous. Should I get tested?"

Never one simply to answer "yes" or "no" when a fuller explanation is possible, I launched into the background on testing. As a nurse, Randi was interested in my detailed explanation, and as my sister, she was used to it.

I explained to her that there are two main tests used to diagnose Covid-19: PCR testing and antigen testing. But before I went into the details on each of these, I told her that it was important to understand the testing concepts of *sensitivity* and *specificity*.

In medical school, we all took a brief course in epidemiology, the study of the incidence, distribution, and control of diseases. The course lacks the blood and guts of other courses and covers material foreign, and of no particular interest, to most medical students. We don't take it very seriously, unfortunately. Buried in this short epidemiology course is a very brief discussion of sensitivity and specificity. I was more intrigued than most of my fellow students by these concepts, but I didn't fully grasp their significance until residency.

My residency director, Dr. Braham, believed that to be a really good diagnostician and clinician, you not only needed to understand both of these concepts, but you needed to live with them in the daily practice of medicine. This was never truer than in the middle of the Covid-19 pandemic.

The s*ensitivity* of a test tells us the *accuracy of positive test results*. During medical school, to help us remember this for an exam, we memorized this as sensitivity = PID (positive in disease). For example, cardiac catheterization (when you inject dye into the heart and use an X-ray to see if there is any arterial blockage) results are 100 percent sensitive; if a patient has heart disease, this will always show up on the cardiac catheterization results. In medical terms, a 100 percent sensitive test is called the "Gold Standard." The term "Gold Standard" dates back to the 1800s and early 1900s, when every U.S. dollar was backed by gold. For physicians, the Gold Standard is a test that gives a clear and indisputable diagnosis of a condition or disease.

Most tests are not 100 percent sensitive. For example, a stress test is another type of test used to diagnose coronary disease.

During a stress test, the patient wears a monitor and exercises on a treadmill with increasing levels of intensity. The physician watches the monitor for signs of coronary artery disease displayed as changes on the electrocardiogram. Typical stress tests have, at best, a sensitivity of 80 percent; 20 percent of the time, they will give a false negative and indicate that the patient does not have coronary artery disease when, in fact, they do.

So why would we ever use a stress test to check for heart disease instead of a test with higher sensitivity, such as a cardiac catheterization? For two reasons: cardiac catheterization comes with greater risk (although the test is relatively safe and we do not see many complications, it is riskier than a stress test) and greater cost.

The *specificity* of a test is the *accuracy of negative test results*. In medical school, we are taught that specificity = NIH (negative in health). This measures how often the test is *negative* and correctly indicates that a patient is healthy.

One could say that a cardiac catheterization, in addition to being 100 percent sensitive, also is 100 percent specific because, if it is negative, we can be sure that the patient does not have coronary artery disease. Stress tests, on the other hand, have a specificity in the range of 70-80 percent – meaning that 20-30 percent of the time the test will be positive despite the patient actually not having coronary artery disease – a false positive.

At this point in my explanation, Randi broke in. “Can we cut to the chase? Are there any tests that are 100 percent accurate for Covid-19?”

“No,” I responded, before continuing with Epidemiology 101.

Physicians rely on patient histories and exams to determine pre-test probability, which is the likelihood that a patient has the disease prior to performing a diagnostic test. Absent a Gold Standard test, a physician will use a patient’s pre-test probability, in combination with the test result, to determine if the patient has the disease.

A good clinician does a test to confirm what they already know – not to go on a fishing expedition. If a patient complains of pain in his chest that radiates down his arm when he climbs stairs and that goes away within a minute of reaching the top step, the attending doctor will ask about family history: do close relatives have coronary artery disease, high blood pressure, or high cholesterol? If the answer is yes to all of those questions, then even a first-year medical student would know that there is a high pre-test probability of the patient having coronary artery disease. If this patient with a high pre-test probability has a positive stress test, even with a sensitivity of only 80 percent, it is extremely likely that the patient has coronary artery disease. On the other hand, if his stress test is negative this would be concerning as a possible false negative. In this situation a good clinician might skip over the stress test and go right to a cardiac catheterization.

Usually, test results are in line with expectations. I gave Randi two Covid-19 examples:

- For a patient with a high pre-test probability (for example, a patient who just returned from China or Spain in March and has symptoms) and a positive Covid-19 test result, the physician can be confident that the patient has the disease.
- For a patient with a low pre-test probability (for example, a patient with no symptoms and no known exposure to Covid-19) and a negative test, the physician can be confident that the patient does not have the disease.

The real challenge for a physician, I explained, is when results are *not* in line with expectations.

- A patient has a high pre-test probability (for example, a patient who has Covid-19 symptoms and a spouse with a positive test result) but gets a negative result. This is tricky. The physician needs to consider, and probably even conclude, that they are dealing with a false negative (a result that indicates the patient does not have the disease when they actually do). This was a common occurrence during the first wave of Covid-19.

- A patient has a low pre-test probability (for example, a patient who has no symptoms, no identified risk, and who has been social distancing aggressively), but gets a positive test result. This is *really* tricky. The physician needs to consider the possibility of a false positive result that indicates the patient has the disease when actually they do not. This problem often arises when you do widespread screening of a group, such as thousands of college kids returning to campus, with a test that is not that sensitive. In reality, it is difficult to ignore any positive results during a pandemic because doing so would put others at risk. But it is likely that many of these positive results are just wrong.

Physicians assess patients for the likelihood of various diseases on a daily basis. While no doctor does a formal mathematical analysis of sensitivity, specificity, and pre-test probability, a good decision maker keeps these concepts constantly in mind when making choices about patient care.

I apologized for the long-winded prelude but told Randi that these concepts are key to understanding the problems and challenges of testing for Covid-19.

I then explained that, for Covid-19, tests look for the presence of the virus, either through its genetic code (RNA) for polymerase chain reaction (PCR) testing, or through the presence of one of the unique proteins on the surface of the virus, referred to as antigen testing.

The PCR test requires a sample that is typically obtained by pushing a long swab way up the nasal-pharyngeal cavity (you get a swab so far up your nose that it reaches the top of your throat). One patient described it as "tickling the back of your eyeballs." You can alternatively test the nasal cavity, saliva, or blood, but these results have a lower sensitivity or specificity than swabs of the nasal-pharyngeal cavity. Scientists currently are working on more reliable tests that use a simple nasal swab or saliva sample so that patients can avoid the discomfort of getting their nasal-pharyngeal cavity swabbed.

Some experts have suggested that a better place from which to get a sample is the anus. This made sense to us, as we were seeing increasing numbers of patients with diarrhea. But our nursing staff correctly felt that most patients would rather do the nasal-pharyngeal swab. One patient was convinced that he had Covid-19 and came for a test – it came back negative. A few days later, he was sicker, with all the typical Covid-19 symptoms. He wanted another test – again, negative. We sent him home, as he was not sick enough for admission, and told him to quarantine. When he came in a third time, I suggested that the nurse do an anal swab. When presented with the choice, he left and did not come back for further testing.

For the PCR test, a technician takes the sample and places it in a vial, then puts it in a PCR machine. The machine, with the assistance of chemicals called reagents, looks for presence of Covid-19 RNA and converts it to DNA. Then, it replicates the DNA. Now, with a large quantity of Covid-19 DNA in the sample, the disease is easily identified (if it is present). The PCR test takes between two and four hours.

In early March 2020, the CDC had to approve every test before we could send the sample to be analyzed. At this point, we did not have the capability to do our own testing at the hospital, nor were local labs equipped to do so.

As was widely reported, there were problems with the CDC's initial PCR testing. The CDC decided not to use the available WHO tests and, instead, developed its own.

This may have been born out of old-fashioned, American, we-can-do-it-better hubris (and we'll never know whether another presidential administration would have used WHO tests), though, to its credit, prior to Covid-19 the CDC was seen as the international leader in the field of infectious disease. But despite the reputation and expertise of the organization, the initial tests produced by the CDC were contaminated and unusable. It set back our testing efforts in the U.S. considerably; we lost critical weeks – and lives – because of this and have been playing catch up ever since.

Because of the CDC testing failure, requests outpaced available tests. (Even if we had had a good test from the start, the number of available tests may not have kept up with the number of requests – but it would have been significantly better.) As a result, the CDC implemented specific prerequisites for testing.

To get a test, you had to meet all of the following criteria:

1. Recent travel to a country with an active outbreak (China, France, Italy, or Spain) or contact with someone with known Covid-19.
2. Be experiencing symptoms.
3. Have negative results for other infections (e.g., flu).

On the surface, this last requirement might make sense to anyone outside of the medical field. If a patient tested positive for any other disease, we were not permitted to test for Covid-19. But it was clear to everyone working the frontlines that this was flawed thinking. Patients can be infected with two diseases (e.g., you can have the flu and Covid-19 at the same time). In fact, being infected with one might wear down your immune system, making you more susceptible to the other. We were incredulous about this guidance; it was just bad medicine.

These testing restrictions were put in place with the goal of increasing a patient's pre-test probability, but the requirements clearly were driven by the fact that there were just not enough tests to go around. Community spread had taken root – and the restrictions on testing were limiting, counterproductive, and clearly not based on good science or medicine.

Early in the pandemic, the CDC would take days to approve our requests to test patients who met all of the criteria. When it finally did grant approval, we did not get the results for an additional one to two weeks – and, in some cases, we never received results at all.

You can see the problem. We were running blindfolded with scissors in both hands. Because we didn't receive results for weeks at a time, we had to treat all of our suspected Covid-19 patients as positive, increasing the demand for PPE and specialized rooms and increasing stress for patients and staff. And when we did receive results, the information was barely useful because so much time had elapsed between the test and the result.

The lack of testing meant that some people with undiagnosed Covid-19 continued with their normal routines, interacting with others in the community and spreading the disease. Restricting testing to only those with symptoms also masked the number of asymptomatic carriers of Covid-19. Even though the CDC testing guidelines were so strict, the government clearly understood that asymptomatic carriers of Covid-19 could transmit the disease. This is why everyone entering the White House or coming into contact with the President was tested, regardless of symptoms.

When a higher number of tests became available and the CDC loosened its testing guidelines, the pent-up demand meant that the testing capacity was again overwhelmed. Thankfully, the situation improved when commercial laboratories started to analyze tests. When we heard that LabCorp, a company that operates more clinical labs than any other company in the world, was able to perform tests on the West Coast, we contacted them and made arrangements to start overnighting tests to them. We received results back in three to five days, which was a big help. But as word got out, that facility also became overwhelmed, and it took longer to get results again. The same thing happened when LabCorp began testing at an east coast facility; the situation initially improved, but the lab quickly became overwhelmed and the results were once again delayed.

Finally, we arranged to send our testing to a small lab just over the state border in Rockland County, New York. That lab consistently sent us results in 24 to 48 hours. This was an enormous help. But to complicate matters, since we were suddenly able to conduct a much larger number of tests, Holy Name came dangerously close to running out of testing swabs and media (the liquid the swab is placed in). Luckily, our Lab Director, Ed Torres, was able to synthesize a substitute for the media.

Though we were glad to now have timely test results, we were very concerned about the accuracy of both the CDC tests and the commercial tests. Neither the CDC nor the commercial labs gave us details about the testing accuracy. They simply told us that the test was "effective." But "effective" is a term that means different things to different people.

I read an interesting survey back in medical school. The surveyor asked scientists and politicians to put a number on the probability that an event would occur if it was described as "likely," "probable," or "almost certain." For example, if a ball pulled out of a hat was "likely" to be red, how many times out of 10 would it actually be red? There was a huge gap between the scientists and the politicians. Politicians thought something that was "likely" to occur probably happened nine times out of 10. In contrast, the scientists put the number closer to just over five times out of 10.

Suppose I asked the readers of this book to guess how often an "effective" test would produce a false positive or false negative. I suspect the answers would vary greatly. If I asked a group of physicians the same question, the range of answers might be narrower, but it would still vary considerably.

To determine what "effective" meant in actuality, Dr. Drew Olsen, our Chief of Pathology, asked the commercial labs for a more precise definition. He learned, to our consternation, that in their rush to develop a test, the labs had not done the analysis that would allow them to determine accuracy. We discussed this concern on our daily calls with the other hospitals. When we pooled our data, we reached the consensus that PCR testing for Covid-19 seemed to have a sensitivity and specificity in the 80-90 percent range (but this was just an educated guess). With a sensitivity of 80 percent, 20 out of every 100 people who have the disease are going to be told their test is negative when, in fact, they have Covid-19.

In the middle of a pandemic, deciding how to treat these likely false negatives was an easy call. If a patient had symptoms consistent with Covid-19 and needed to be admitted to the hospital, even if their test result was negative, we assumed it was a false negative and treated them for Covid-19. It did however, result in tough conversations with patients, telling them that although their results were negative, we thought they were infected. But as the prevalence of disease and the average pre-test probability dropped after the first wave of the pandemic, we had daily conversations about this group of patients and had to make clinical judgements as to whether to treat them as having Covid-19 or not.

We faced a potentially larger problem with patients who tested negative and had symptoms, but who were not sick enough to be admitted to the hospital. Given the false comfort of receiving a negative test when in reality they had

Covid-19, patients might refuse to quarantine or be less careful about social distancing and, in lowering their guard, infect others and increase community spread.

Recent autopsy studies may give us a clue as to why the false negative rate for PCR testing is so high. In these studies, Covid-19 was found throughout deceased patients' bodies, but in some of these patients, it was absent in the nasal passageway. Are these the subset of patients where we have false negatives, and would it decrease the false negatives if we instead tested stool or blood? Further studies will hopefully shed some light on this possibility.

In early April, with FDA approval, Holy Name, like most other hospitals, was able to obtain reagents to perform our own in-house testing with rapid turnaround. We already had a PCR machine in-house that had been used to identify other viruses and bacteria. With new reagents, it could test for Covid-19. Different models of PCR machines use different reagents, and I worried that there would be a shortage of reagents if we only had one type of PCR machine. To hedge our bets, we bought three new PCR machines from three different vendors at $225,000 apiece. Not an inexpensive decision, but well worth the cost.

By July 2020, Holy Name had four PCR machines for in-house use, running pretty much full time. As Covid-19 broke out in other parts of the country, the demand for reagents skyrocketed, as I had predicted. We added reagents for our four different machines to the list of supplies we inventoried on a daily basis to ensure that we didn't run out.

Widespread testing in other countries allowed government and medical officials to pinpoint hot spots, conduct effective contact tracing, and quarantine individuals as warranted. They got control of the virus. In the U.S., we allowed it to run rampant. The availability of early testing might not have stopped the pandemic, but looking at what happened in other countries certainly leads me to believe that it would have greatly lessened the initial spread and reduced the number of hospitalizations and deaths.

At this point, my sister again broke in, frustrated with my long-winded answer. “Adam, just tell me, should I get a test?”

Only the PCR test was available at the time and although sensitivity and specificity were far from perfect, I said, “Yes, get tested. But no matter the results, you need to quarantine. A negative test will make you less stressed, but just in case, stay away from others. And if you get a positive test, don’t panic. Just monitor for symptoms and stay away from others.”

“So, get tested, stay calm, and no matter what, stay away from others? You could have led with that.”

**On August 22, 2020**

- More than 175,000 Covid-19 deaths in the U.S.
- Two dozen cases in three states are linked to the Sturgis Motorcycle rally.
- New Hampshire allows restaurants to open indoors at 100 percent capacity.

CHAPTER FOURTEEN

# "Went to a Garden Party…" Learned my Lesson Well?

*"It was a serious failure for me, as a public figure,*
*to go maskless at the Whitehouse.*
*I am lucky to be alive."*

**Chris Christie**
Former Governor of New Jersey
October 21, 2020

On September 26, 2020, approximately 200 people, including some of the most powerful people in the world, gathered in the White House Rose Garden to celebrate the announcement of the new Supreme Court nominee. All attendees were required to have a negative Covid-19 test. I don't think it's an exaggeration to say that these attendees had better access to Covid-19 testing than anyone else in America. During the event, the group packed closely together, many did not wear masks, and hugs and handshakes were the norm. The outdoor Rose Garden announcement was followed by an indoor reception.

More than 30 infections have been traced to that event, including President Trump, First Lady Melania Trump, former Governor of New Jersey Chris Christie, senators, journalists, and White House staff. Several of those infected required hospitalization.

This is a warning: do not become complacent as testing becomes more available. Covid-19 testing, as we have learned, still is just not that accurate. All it takes is one false negative to lead to lax social distancing measures, to then reate a super-spreader event.

* * * * *

In early May, the FDA authorized emergency use of antigen testing different than PCR testing), the type of testing used at the White House. Instead of looking for viral RNA, antigen testing looks for Covid-19 unique proteins on he surface of the virus.

Antigen testing for Covid-19 was used extensively outside of the U.S. and could be done in a doctor's office or even at home. As with PCR testing, ntigen testing typically starts with a swab from the back of the nose or throat. nitial Covid-19 antigen tests resembled a home pregnancy test and gave results within 15 minutes. Now, testing centers have machines that can run multiple tests simultaneously.

Starting in April, before antigen tests were even approved in the U.S., numerous resellers (companies that buy equipment overseas and then resell them n the U.S. market) approached me about buying antigen testing kits. We evaluated many of these kits. For the most part, Drew felt that the quality of these ests was not adequate for our usage. The companies were unknown, they were not willing to provide information on accuracy, and the results were hard to nterpret.

We did get a lead on 2,000 antigen tests that we could import from a eliable German company and that Drew felt were accurate enough and easy to nterpret. Given the dire state of testing, we considered importing these tests, although they were not FDA-approved. The inability to get accurate, reliable, and ast test results was hampering Holy Name's – and the nation's – ability to espond effectively to Covid-19. We felt that during this declared state of emergency, we should proceed with the tests from Germany as long as they were of high quality. However, Don convinced me that pursuing these tests was a folly. He was sure that without FDA approval, the tests would be held up or seized at the border.

Antigen testing, while fast, will always suffer from lower accuracy than PCR testing. Unlike PCR testing, antigen tests do not replicate the virus's RNA. Therefore, antigen tests provide false negatives more frequently than PCR testing mainly because the amount of the virus present in the sample is lower.

Initial antigen testing for Covid-19 had a sensitivity and specificity as low as 50 percent – as accurate as a coin flip. Later antigen tests were reported to be 80-90 percent accurate. However, I still had concerns. These tests' accuracy was evaluated using a small sample of patients who showed symptoms and who therefore likely had a high viral load. I didn't know if the tests would be as accurate when performed on people without symptoms or with smaller viral loads.

We chose not to use antigen testing at the hospital once it was available and FDA-approved, although we continue to assess the viability of these tests and hope to use them in the future on patients with high pre-test probability. Once we had access to adequate PCR testing, we were willing to take the longer result time (two to four hours, compared to 15 minutes) in exchange for greater accuracy.

As antigen testing rolled out in the U.S., it created problems with a significant number of false positives. A notable example was Ohio Governor Mike DeWine, who, despite having a low pre-test probability, tested positive with an antigen test prior to a meeting with the President. Based on the test result, he missed the meeting. However, a follow up PCR test was negative, essentially ruling out Covid-19 when considered with his low pre-test probability.

* * * * *

Screening, a form of testing done in a large population of asymptomatic people, for Covid-19 can be an important tool. Widespread screening can help us detect the presence of a disease in a certain population early, giving us the best chance to catch asymptomatic carriers and limit their exposure to others.

For widespread screening of any disease to be effective:

1. The disease needs to have a high prevalence in the population you are screening. (Check: Covid-19 was running rampant.)
2. The test has to be widely available, relatively inexpensive, and have a rapid turnaround. (Check: antigen testing met those criteria, even if PCR testing did not.)
3. Early diagnosis must lead to action that has an impact on the spread of the disease. (Check: Covid-19-positive patients can quarantine and not infect others.)
4. The test must have a relatively high sensitivity and specificity. (Check with PCR testing, but no check with antigen testing. When we use antigen testing, we undoubtedly will inform screened patients that they are positive when they are not, and we will tell screened patients that they are negative when they are not.)

I remain a strong proponent of screening, accompanied by good education so that patients understand the implications of their test results. However, we need to accept the reality of false readings. And, of course, we need to continue to work toward improving testing to increase sensitivity and specificity.

* * * * *

There is a third type of test associated with Covid-19 – antibody tests. When faced with an intruder, the body produces different types of antibodies to combat the disease. While the PCR and the antigen test look for actual virus (in the form of RNA or proteins), the antibody test looks for the body's response to the disease. We typically test for the presence of these antibodies not to see if you *are* infected, but to see if you *were* infected.

Following an infection, the first antibodies that the body produces are IgM antibodies. They appear early in an infection, and then typically fade away over time. An IgM test can be used as a diagnostic test for certain infectious diseases, such as hepatitis A. Currently, scientists are working on understanding the IgM response for Covid-19 infections to develop a blood test that may help us diagnose Covid-19 in its early stages.

A little later into the infection, the body produces IgG antibodies. IgG antibodies remain in the body longer after the initial infection than IgM antibodies. How long depends on the disease, the individual, and the severity of the infection.

IgG testing for Covid-19 requires a blood sample and has a sensitivity of between 90 and 98 percent. A PCR test reports out as a simple positive or negative result; the antibody test reports out as a value that indicates the level of antibodies in your system.

There are two ways white blood cells, called lymphocytes, help the body to fight intruders. One type of lymphocytes called "B-cells," produce IgM and IgG antibodies, which fight pathogens in the body. Immunity caused by these antibodies is called "B-cell" or "humoral" immunity.

The second type of lymphocyte, T-cells, attacks pathogens directly rather than creating antibodies. Immunity related to these lymphocytes is called "T-cell" or "cellular" immunity. This type of immunity is much more difficult to test for because there are no antibodies to indicate its presence. Scientists hypothesize that cellular immunity may play a larger role in Covid-19 immunity than originally thought, but far more work needs to be done to better understand the body's immune response to Covid-19 and how long it lasts.

On April 21, 2020, at around 3:00 p.m., my assistant, Marisol De La Paz, handed me a stack of antibody test results for the Holy Name staff. I was dreading the results, fearful that the protective measures we had implemented might not have kept our staff safe. I thought that we might have a number of staff that, unbeknown to us or them, were infected but asymptomatic. We didn't. In fact, none of the critical care physicians had positive antibodies, and only a few of the nurses did.

I was a bit surprised that we did not have more staff who had been infected. But my surprise – and relief – was quickly followed by disappointment. I certainly was pleased that the negative pressure rooms, masks, and social distancing worked, and I was thankful that our staff hadn't spread the disease to their families or the larger community. But I realized that a small part of me had hoped that a large number of the staff had had mild cases and were now immune. But that just was not the case. Approximately 15 percent of our staff tested positive for the Covid-19 antibody, consistent with what was being seen in the general local population.

My test results were at the bottom of Marisol's stack. I was expecting it to be positive, convinced that I had had a mild case of Covid-19 before we had been on the lookout for symptoms. But no, it was negative. My coughing and runny nose had probably been just your ordinary, everyday cold.

Again, I was a little disappointed at my test results. I had hoped that I, too, had had a mild infection, recovered, and could worry less going forward. In fact, I may have had Covid-19 (although not likely), but the antibodies may have dissipated by the time I was tested. Either way, I cannot count on having protective immunity.

Not surprisingly, many people who treated Covid-19 patients were convinced they had Covid-19 when they did not. This is a phenomenon I have seen throughout my career – healthcare providers thinking they were ill with a disease, especially an infectious disease, that they had been studying or treating in close quarters. The stress of the situation can lead to somatic symptoms consistent with the illness.

Throughout the next few weeks, we retested all staff who had had an initial positive antibody test to see if their antibody levels remained stable or changed in any way. We found that for many, their antibody levels fell rather quickly, indicating both that the window for verifying a previous infection might be small, and that post-infection immunity might not last indefinitely. But clearly more research needs to be done to fully understand this.

* * * * *

I have noticed recently that medical experts on television are referring to the PCR test as the "Gold Standard." I disagree with this characterization. The Gold Standard is *the* definitive test; it should never be wrong. Experts should not use the phrase "Gold Standard" for PCR testing just because it's the best and most reliable test that we have. It can still be wrong. Next-generation PCR testing likely will have an accuracy level as high as 97-98 percent. However, these next-generation tests still are not widely available and, of more concern, even a test that is 98 percent accurate will still be wrong hundreds of thousands of times when testing tens of millions of people.

As we return (or try to return) to normal, accurate rapid testing will be critical for determining who can go to work, who can go back to school, or who can see the President. But we cannot overwhelm the system again. In addition, even if we have adequate testing available, we need to thoroughly understand the implications of inherently imperfect testing on our policymaking and healthcare lecisions.

**On September 1, 2020**

- More than six million Covid-19 cases and 184,000 Covid-19 deaths in the U.S.
- Colleges and universities have reported 25,000 Covid-19 cases in 37 states.
- A National Institute of Health (NIH) panel recommends against standard use of convalescent plasma for Covid-19 patients until more research is done.
- In Quebec City, 30 cases of Covid-19 are linked to a karaoke bar.

CHAPTER FIFTEEN

# Running a Hospital in the Time of Covid

*"Running a hospital during Covid was intense. Hospitals always deal with decisions of life and death but never before have I been in a situation where so many decisions needed to be made in such a short period of time – and which affected the lives of so many people – staff and patients alike."*

**Mike Maron**
CEO and President, Holy Name Medical Center
September 2, 2020

Running a hospital is never easy. It's like juggling half a dozen balls at once. Running a hospital at the epicenter of Covid-19 was like juggling a dozen flaming knives – that had been greased.

Decisions had to be made at a pace that did not allow for our usual deliberation and collaboration. We needed to be more efficient than ever. Information had to reach top-level management quickly, management had to make decisions nearly instantaneously, and those decisions needed to be communicated back to the rest of the hospital as soon as possible.

We also needed to fill a gap on our leadership team. A few months prior to Covid-19, our long-serving CNO, Sheryl Slonim, had retired. Rather than filling the position immediately, Mike had wanted to try out a new leadership model for our nursing team.

He set up two interdisciplinary committees, one focusing on clinical issues and the other on non-clinical operational issues. The committees were tasked with guiding policy, improving quality of care, and creating operational efficiencies. While this was an interesting model that, in normal times, might have been successful, decision-making by committee during Covid-19 was not practical.

In stepped Michele Acito. Michele is an exceedingly smart nurse practitioner who had spent the last several years running our cardiac and neurological programs. She had leadership experience, and just as importantly, she gets how hospitals work.

Michele arrives at work at 6:30 a.m. every day – one of the few people who consistently shows up before I do. She does whatever it takes to get the job done. She has strong convictions, and is good both with the facts and people.

Michele's ability to think on her feet and to make tough, reasoned choices shone during Covid-19. She was named CNO midway through the first wave. At that time, the operational leadership team was composed of Michele, Mike, Steve, Cedar, and me.

Michele and I worked side by side throughout the pandemic. We were at the hospital every day for 48 straight days in March and April. When we finally could take part of a weekend off, she insisted that I take the Saturday off and she would take the Sunday. She now enjoys telling people that she worked one more day in a row than I did.

During those two months, the sheer number of problems and decisions facing the hospital was astounding. The leadership team delegated authority to all managers to make decisions that under normal circumstances, they might run up the chain of command for input or confirmation. This was the only way to maintain the day-to-day operations of the hospital.

Despite access to state-of-the-art technology, I realized early on that the best way to track patients and resources was the old-fashioned way: by hand. I took a page from my days as Assistant Chief Resident, when I had been responsible for the "bed board," and had whiteboards installed in my office to track all our Covid-19 patients.

Marisol converted my office into a war room. Down came the posters of national parks and photos of my family and up went the whiteboards – everywhere. On these whiteboards, we tracked patients and equipment. They displayed the status of every bed in the hospital: which ones were occupied by Covid-19 patients, which ones were Covid-19-patient-ready, and which ones were not. Every occupied bed was marked with a Covid-19 patient's initials, age, number of days in the ICU, number of days on a ventilator, and a patient assessment to help us determine expected survivability. This last point may seem harsh, but it was critical to evaluating needs for the following day or days. Along the bottom of one of the boards, we noted how many ventilators, gloves, and masks we had available.

Every time we looked at the boards, we could quickly assess the numbers and our needs. But we also saw the initials, a stark reminder that these were not just numbers, but people – and that their lives hinged on the decisions we made. Several times a day, our leadership team would gather, each in a separate corner of my office, survey the boards, decide which patients to transfer from one unit to another, adjust staffing, and review supply needs.

Throughout the day, Marisol would review and update the whiteboards. She is reassuringly competent, unflappable, and efficient; that's what makes her such a great assistant. Although Marisol never had any direct contact with our patients, she often had tears in her eyes as she wiped away initials on the boards. Covid-19 was tough on everyone at the hospital, not just the medical staff.

Our daily department heads meetings were tightly run and never more than 30 minutes. Emma Yamada, our Director of Data Science, would start these meetings with a census-like summary of our Covid-19 patients, something like:

"We have 18 critical patients on ventilators, 45 admitted non-ICU patients, and another 24 in the ED. In total, we have tested 485 patients and are awaiting results for 251 of them." Each member of the team would then report on their area and raise any issue they were having so that we could brainstorm solutions. At the end of each meeting, everyone knew exactly what needed to be accomplished in the next 24 hours so that we could stay ahead of the wave.

One day, Emma finished her Covid-19 report with a twist. "And the word of the day is 'acnestis.'" She then read the word's definition (the part of an animal's skin that it cannot reach to scratch, usually the space between the shoulder blades). She added it to an electronic whiteboard that also tracked census and supply data. The word of the day was a hit. Emma chose a new word for every meeting. Soon, everyone tried to include the word of the day in that day's report – not always easy on the spot and with words like "trenchant" (vigorous or incisive in expression or style), "pandiculation" (a stretching and stiffening, especially of the trunk and extremities, such as right after waking up), or "quire" (four sheets of paper or parchment folded to form eight leaves, as in medieval manuscripts). It injected a little levity into very hard and emotionally draining days. And, yes, "quire" is extremely tough to work into a medical report in 2020.

At one meeting, Nancy Palamara, our Director of Pharmacy, indicated that, on top of shortages of PPE, tests, and ventilators, she was also concerned about drug shortages. We had far more patients than usual who required similar medications, and several patients in the ICU who required massive quantities of paralytics, narcotics, and sedatives. Nancy was concerned that we were going to run out. She proposed that she work with a group of physicians to determine potential substitutes for these drugs that we could use if the shortage got worse. They developed this backup plan, but Nancy scrambled to keep ahead, contacting other hospitals and suppliers. Because of her efforts, we never had to resort to this substitution plan – but we were prepared.

During this time, intra-hospital communication was critical. Immediately following our daily management meeting at Holy Name, Michele and I had our daily video call with the CMOs and CNOs of the other Northern New Jersey hospitals. We would convene in her office and take our regular seats, she at her desk and I six feet behind her in a leather chair. She had large pictures of flowers on her walls, often matched by real flowers sitting on a round conference table that her husband had sent.

On the calls, the hospitals developed a rhythm detailing their daily reports: how many known Covid-19 patients they had, how many patients with results pending, how many they thought had false negative test results, and how many patients were on ventilators. While Holy Name's daily meeting was all about coming up with action plans, this call was about learning what was happening at other hospitals and sharing knowledge we had gained.

These calls included daily discussions on masks, gowns, and ventilators. When possible, we arranged to share our supplies. We also shared insights such as information regarding increased clotting, the reality of the significant volume of false negative results, and information regarding treatments. Were steroids making a difference? What about plasma or hydroxychloroquine? We didn't have good studies to rely upon, so we hoped to make better decisions for all of our patients by pooling our anecdotal results.

While some competition among hospitals is inevitable, I hope that we can learn from this experience, and that there will be a little more cooperation in the healthcare industry post-Covid-19. It would be good for patients.

One of the best examples of cooperation in the medical field prior to Covid-19 was the existence of peer-reviewed medical journals. These journals are the main method by which the medical community effectively disseminates best medical practices. They are how medical professionals keep abreast of new treatments, the most recent studies, and breakthrough innovations. The journals (for the most part) ensure academic rigor, vigorous review, and the opportunity for others to replicate results. It is a good system. But it takes time.

During the pandemic, we did not have time to wait for journal articles; patients were walking through our doors and needed to be treated immediately. While community spread of information was helpful, and sometimes even critical, it was not always enough. I should not have needed to depend on the good intentions of a fellow doctor to learn about blood clots caused by Covid-19. That should have been reported to a central database, confirmed through autopsies, and quickly conveyed to healthcare providers nationwide. Delaying communication of such essential information by even a few days could result in lost lives.

Our profession needs to think about how we can better disseminate information during emergencies. We should not leave it up to elected officials. Numerous physician organizations can take the lead on this instead, such as the American Medical Association (AMA) and the American College of Physicians (ACP).

These organizations could create websites that are only accessible to licensed physicians in good standing. These physicians could post their anecdotal experiences, which would be subject to a review process. This system would not seek to eliminate reasonable findings, but to quickly screen out suggestions that make no sense or are potentially dangerous. It would have to be clear that these anecdotal experiences were not evidence-based. However, with a new disease, pooled anecdotes could be a useful tool until there is enough evidence-based research on which to base treatment.

* * * * *

Following the first wave of Covid-19, we made some changes in the way we operate. We significantly changed the logistics of registration and patient flow into and around the hospital to keep patients as separate from each other as possible.

All patients are now registered over the phone, and this registration includes a telephonic screening for symptoms of Covid-19. We refer any patient with concerning symptoms to our telemedicine program so that we can take appropriate next actions, which may include delaying a scheduled test or procedure and/or arranging for Covid-19 testing.

We created separate entrances into the hospital based on what service patients needed. Patients going into radiology entered in one location, patients scheduled for outpatient surgery went into another, and so on. At all entrances, patients were temperature-screened with special computer monitors that also reminded patients to wear their masks, which we required for all people entering the hospital. We spread out the scheduling of patient appointments and limited the number of patients in each waiting area so that patients and staff could socially distance.

By mid-August, we no longer required staff to wear N95 masks for all patient interactions. Instead, staff wore surgical masks unless they were working with a known or suspected patient with Covid-19.

We gradually began to allow visitors again for non-Covid-19 patients. This was a major discussion point among Holy Name's leadership. Initially, we all were reluctant to allow visitation, as we had real concerns that this could trigger increased spread. Ultimately, we weighed the risk of spread against the benefits of allowing visitors. Not only do visitors assist in recovery, but some patients were refusing to schedule needed procedures because they wanted family or friends there to support them. We decided to allow one visitor for patients undergoing surgery and later allowed one visitor at a time for all non-Covid-19 admitted patients. More recently, we have allowed key volunteers to return, as well as some student observers. We monitor the incidence of community spread and reevaluate these policies regularly.

* * * * *

At a board of directors meeting at a typical hospital, the board will spend 90 percent of the meeting talking about finances and less than 10 percent talking about medical issues.

At Holy Name, the board of trustees begins every meeting by discussing a specific patient and the care they received. The case is chosen to illustrate a patient care issue that management wants to bring to the board's attention. But the board also spends a fair share of its time making sure the hospital's financial situation is sound.

Patients are our priority, but hospitals are businesses – big businesses. Ryan Kennedy, our CFO, likes to remind me of the old hospital saying: "No margin, no mission." To offer services to the community and provide the best possible care to the greatest number of people, we need to make sure that our finances are stable. Poor financial decisions on our part will impact the quality and accessibility of care in the community. This is the reality that all hospitals must deal with.

Medical equipment is expensive; an MRI machine costs more than $1.5 million. But cost is just one of many factors that hospitals consider when making a large purchase. Is the equipment replacing old technology? Will it improve the quality of care we offer? How often will we be able to use the equipment? (We don't like expensive equipment sitting idle.) And, of course, what is the cost and reimbursement related to use of the equipment? These questions have to be asked and answered to keep hospitals financially healthy.

Covid-19 strained the finances of hospitals on many fronts. Put simply, costs shot up and revenues plummeted. We were hit with a steep decline in elective surgeries and procedures such as colonoscopies, hip and knee replacements, and hernia repairs. Before Covid-19, more than 50 percent of our revenues came from such outpatient services. These bread-and-butter services went to zero almost overnight – creating real financial challenges.

Holy Name, like most hospitals that faced Covid-19, received a significant cash infusion from the Coronavirus Aid, Relief, and Economic Security (CARES) Act, the first Covid-19 federal assistance bill. Without this assistance, Holy Name and many other hospitals would have struggled to keep their doors open. The CARES money was critical in allowing us not to lay off a single employee or reduce salaries. Whether there will be additional CARES money for Covid-19 is unclear at this moment.

Although healthcare costs are a constant topic of discussion and debate in the U.S., not many people know how health insurance and hospital finances actually work. In the 1980s, the federal government implemented a rule affecting hospital finances that is still in place today. Hospitals don't get reimbursed by Medicare or private insurance companies for every little thing they do. Instead, they get reimbursed at a set price for a given procedure or diagnosis, called a diagnostic related group (DRG). For instance, a knee replacement, bleeding ulcer, or pneumonia each has its own DRG associated with a standard reimbursement.

Let's look at a patient admitted with pneumonia. Hospitals get paid the same amount for a relatively healthy patient with pneumonia who only requires two or three days of in-patient care as they do for a pneumonia patient with significant underlying medical issues and who requires a much longer hospital stay. This example over-simplifies the payment model a bit, but this is the basic method by which hospitals get paid. In this model, the hospital is paid less than it costs to care for a significant number of its patients. Therefore, it has to be as efficient as possible in all of the care it provides if it is going to remain financially stable.

Early on in the pandemic, there was no DRG for Covid-19. Medicare instructed us to bill these hospital admissions with a relatively low-value, non-specific DRG code. This meant that we received very little reimbursement for the care we provided to early Covid-19 patients. Later on, Medicare created a higher-value, specific DRG code for Covid-19, but as Ryan reminds me on a regular basis, the Covid-19 reimbursement by Medicare and Medicaid still does not fully cover the cost of caring for these very sick patients.

In the U.S., as a result of the CARES Act patients in most cases do not pay a penny for Covid-19 treatment (hospitals do get paid by insurance). There have been some sensationalized stories of individuals with bills for hundreds of thousands of dollars after surviving Covid-19, but those individuals eventually paid nothing.

During the first wave of Covid-19, Holy Name spent more than $1 million to purchase one experimental drug (for which there is no direct reimbursement in the Covid-19 DRG), and more than $1 million washing gowns, building ISO-pods, and creating negative pressure rooms. We also gave well-deserved hazard bonuses to our workers. They were going above and beyond their normal work and putting their lives and the lives of their families on the line to help others. The CARES money will help offset some of these costs and will make up for some of the lost revenue caused by significant reduction in non-Covid-19 patients.

When our financial team discussed Covid-19 expenditures, Ryan would often agree with my thoughts on why we needed to spend money on a certain aspect of Covid-19 care. Other times, he would not. In those cases, we brought the decision to Mike. Ryan would break down why we should avoid or delay the expenditure (as a CFO should) and I would spell out the medical reasons for the purchase. But if I said, "Mike, we need this," he would almost always respond, "Ryan, find the money."

I remind Ryan on a frequent basis that although we have to function like a business, we are a hospital first, and at times are going to make clinical decisions that don't make financial sense. However, while not every single thing we do has to make money, if we operate at a loss, we will not be able to keep our doors open. In healthcare, this is a delicate balancing act. I am glad to say that I never felt pressure to compromise care for Covid-19 patients, or any patients, because of financial constraints, and I know that Holy Name will survive this pandemic.

* * * * *

When any hospital goes out of business, it can be devastating for the community in which it is located. This is especially true for poorer communities – whether in the U.S. or another country. When I joined Holy Name, I learned that it was connected with a hospital located in northern Haiti. The connection between Holy Name and Hôpital Sacré Coeur was initially informal. Several members of our medical staff and the Sisters of St. Joseph of Peace had taken the hospital and its community, the village of Milot, under their wing. After the earthquake of 2010, which strained Hôpital Sacré Coeur's resources to the breaking point, Mike made several trips down to Haiti to see if he personally, and Holy Name as an organization, could be of help. He learned that without sustained help, the hospital was not likely to survive.

Mike came back after one of his trips and told our board and the Sisters that we had no choice but to step in. Our board agreed, and Sacré Coeur became an official part of Holy Name. Now, the Holy Name community includes more than just Northern New Jersey and the New York City area; it also includes Northern Haiti.

We spend more than $1 million per year to help keep Sacré Coeur operating, and our medical staff spends hundreds of hours each year helping improve care for the people of Northern Haiti. Others from the Holy Name team have pitched in, as well. Greg Bozzo, who heads the outside construction team for Holy Name, has spent time at Hôpital Sacré Coeur working on the hospital's buildings and infrastructure. On one trip, while working on the roof of the hospital, he fell, fracturing his pelvis. He was transported first by car for six hours over a bumpy, poorly-repaired (and, therefore, painful) road before being airlifted to Holy Name. It was a harrowing experience. However, he was undeterred and he continues to travel to Haiti.

Mike has traveled to Sacré Coeur close to 50 times, and many of Holy Name's staff have gone down multiple times. When we go, our duffel bags are full of IVs, medications, surgical supplies, and bandages.

I have visited Sacré Coeur five times, working with the Haitian medical staff, helping to establish policies and procedures, and jumping right in to work at the clinic or assist with HIV/AIDS patients. HIV/AIDS is rampant in Haiti, though medicine is provided free to all patients at Sacré Coeur, which helps keep its impact under control.

Sacré Coeur is not just critical to the health of the people of Northern Haiti, but it also is the major employer in the region. For many workers, the meals they eat at the hospital are the only nutritious food they will eat in a given day.

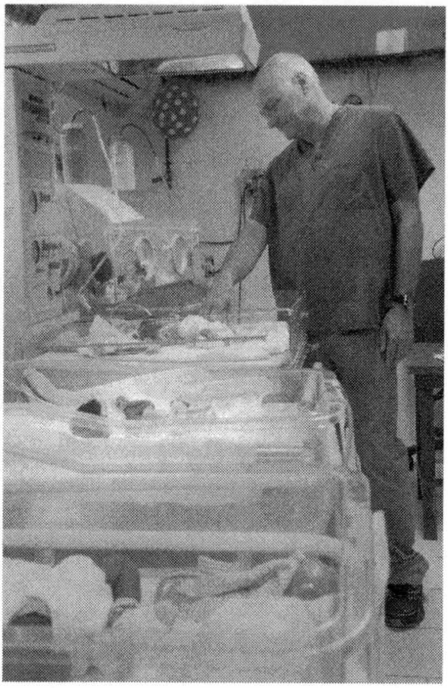

Mike visiting the neonatal-care center in Haiti.

There are people who ask, "Why is Holy Name, a medium-sized hospital in the middle of the most competitive healthcare market in the world, doing this?" Mike just says, "The need is there, and we can make a difference." He also points out that Holy Name benefits from the relationship, as well. "When we send people to Haiti, they are changed. It puts our issues in perspective and draws us together as a team. I would rather send staff to Sacré Coeur, where they can impact lives, than send people to executive trainings."

I am convinced that one of the reasons we fared relatively well in the time of Covid-19 is that our team had great training on how to accomplish a lot with limited resources. It is my strong belief that our commitment and time spent at Hôpital Sacré Coeur prepared the staff at Holy Name to better deal with this pandemic, which required ingenious, innovative thinking and a willingness to explore new ways of getting the job done. We creatively utilized staff and equipment and thought outside the box – as we do in Haiti. Not exactly juggling greased flaming knives, but pretty darn close.

**On September 14, 2020**

- 55 cases of Covid-19 in staff of New York City schools.
- Oxford University vaccine trial resumes after being halted by an unexplained illness in a volunteer.
- Macy's cancels its Thanksgiving Day Parade.

CHAPTER SIXTEEN

# Plenty of Blame to Go Around

*"When there are so many different figures, it can cause real confusion about whom to listen to, or who's in charge of what, and if the response becomes political, it's a disaster, because people won't know if you are making recommendations based on science or politics, and so there's risk they'll start to tune out."*

**Dr. Tom Inglesby**
Director, Center for Health Security
Johns Hopkins University
May 4, 2020

When it comes to this pandemic, there is plenty of blame to go around. But I've never been one to play the blame game. The observations that follow are meant as constructive criticism that hopefully will lead to better decision-making in the future.

China reported the first Covid-19 death in early January 2020 and the first reported death in the U.S. was in Washington State on February 29 – a man who had traveled to Wuhan, China. We later learned, based on an autopsy, that the first Covid-19 death in the U.S. was actually on February 6 in Santa Clara County, California. Holy Name's first wave of known Covid-19 patients came in March.

The federal government, for the most part, wasted this critical time between January and March. The government's errors included:

1. Not getting the federal stockpile of essential PPE and equipment in order – and not adding to it.

2. Failing to establish a federal plan to distribute the stockpile.
3. Failing to adequately develop, secure, and distribute Covid-19 tests.
4. Not having medical experts take the lead in communicating and educating the public.

These missteps severely hampered our ability to attack and contain this disease. These errors are particularly egregious based on an interview in early February with reporter Bob Woodward and President Trump which was released in October. The President was clear – the administration knew that Covid-19 was more deadly than even strenuous flus and potentially airborne, and they still chose not to act and downplayed the risks.

These mistakes were all the more frustrating because other countries got it right. On March 26, New Zealand required a self-quarantine for all but essential workers. Five weeks later, they loosened restrictions, and after a total of seven weeks they lifted the restrictions completely. As of September 11, 2020, New Zealand had reported a total of 1,401 cases (.03 percent of the population) and 22 deaths (.0004 percent of the population). South Korea relied heavily on contact tracing and extensive testing. As of October 27, it had a little more than 26,000 cases (.05 percent of the population) and 460 deaths (.0009 percent of the population). In comparison, as of late October, the U.S. had close to 9 million cases (2.7 percent of the population) and over 230,000 deaths (.07 percent of the population) – arguably the worst numbers of any country in the world.

Several bewildering decisions from the administration contributed to our overall poor performance: disbanding the CDC virus watch outpost in Wuhan; disregarding the pandemic plan put in place by the previous administration; choosing to have elected, non-medical officials give out daily information (or, more accurately, misinformation) rather than an infectious disease or public health expert; and generally not relying on evidence-based medicine.

These failures and decisions cost lives – tens of thousands of lives and counting – and warrant a level of outrage that I have not yet seen from the general public.

Handling a pandemic is a massive challenge, and it's impossible to do so perfectly. But other countries managed to get it right. We need to ask ourselves why we did not.

Now that the election is over, we need to create a nonpartisan panel of medical professionals and former health officials to examine why this went so wrong and what can be done to prepare for the next pandemic. This could be similar to the 9/11 Commission, led by former New Jersey Governor Tom Kean, which looked at government failures surrounding 9/11 in an attempt to prevent future attacks. A Covid-19 panel should not assess blame, but would make sure that we do not repeat these mistakes in the future.

But the first step is admitting that we did poorly, and, as a nation, I do not think we are there yet.

* * * * *

On March 30, 2020, the USNS Comfort, a Navy hospital ship with 1,000 beds and 1,100 medical personnel, traveled from Norfolk, Virginia, up the East Coast to the Hudson River, and docked at Pier 90 in Manhattan. This floating hospital was sent to help relieve the pressure on the New York area's stressed hospitals. It arrived with great fanfare; crowds of New Yorkers defied social distancing protocols and packed the Hudson piers to greet the boat and its crew. Less than one month later, the Comfort departed, having treated less than 200 patients. It was considered a resounding failure by the medical community.

The USNS Comfort was the most visible pop-up hospital (and the biggest pop-up hospital failure), but there were others in the Northern New

Jersey area, most notably the Jacob Javits Convention Center on the West Side of Manhattan, with 1,000 pop-up beds, and the New Jersey Meadowlands Exposition Center in Secaucus, with 250 pop-up beds.

The issue with the pop-ups was that they didn't know and couldn't find their purpose. At first, they were meant to divert non-Covid-19 patients away from over-crowded hospitals. But elective surgeries had stopped when Covid-19 began to spread, and patients did not want to go to a pop-up hospital for delivery of a baby or emergency surgery – understandably. These hospitals lacked the advanced equipment, testing abilities, and full-service pharmacies of established hospitals. They also lacked a strong bench of physicians with specialized expertise that patients might need in an emergency. As a result, there were almost no non-Covid-19 patients for these pop-ups to serve.

Then, pop-ups became overflow centers for Covid-19 patients – but only for patients who were no longer or not yet in critical condition. Many Covid-19 patients who did check in to pop-up hospitals quickly checked out after seeing the facilities.

Additionally, the pop-up hospitals did not have negative pressure rooms, which put their nurses, physician assistants, physicians, and non-Covid-19 patients at risk of contracting Covid-19. It would have been relatively easy to build these facilities with Covid-19 in mind, specifically including dozens of negative pressure rooms for patient isolation. But that didn't happen.

In the future, I would recommend that state and federal officials survey hospitals and provide them with supplies and personnel instead of creating pop-up hospitals. If Holy Name had been asked, "What do you need to expand capacity?" we would have said, "Send trained medical and nursing staff." The staff who worked at the pop-up hospitals would have been more useful if they had been integrated into our team, where they could have quickly learned from our staff who had experience with Covid-19 and treated hundreds of patients.

I could have added as many as 100 additional beds if I had had more staff. It would have required creativity (something my team had in spades), such as maybe converting Holy Name's cafeteria into a Covid-19 ward, but patients in such a location would have had better access to medical resources than those in pop-ups did. Additional staff also would have allowed us to give our overworked and overstressed workers much-needed breaks.

A better use for these pop-up spaces could have been as quarantine centers for patients who no longer needed hospitalization but who could not easily quarantine due to their living situation. Let me be clear: I am not proposing mandated quarantines, as has been done in other countries. But these facilities would have been a reasonable option for patients who no longer needed acute in-patient care but could not safely quarantine at home. For instance, in the New York region, once nursing home patients had recovered, they were released back to the nursing home. In New York alone, more than 6,000 of these patients, some of whom may still have been infectious, were sent back to their facilities.

These potential "pop-up quarantine centers" could have been built with infection control measures including negative pressure isolation rooms, would have been relatively easy to staff, and would have required minimal resources because they would have cared for patients who no longer needed acute care. Quarantine centers would have been an efficient way to reduce community spread and reduce the pressure on hospitals that were full with recovering Covid-19 patients who had nowhere else to go.

* * * * *

I have already mentioned my exasperation with the federal stockpile of emergency materials. You hope you never need a stockpile, and that can lead to a failure to maintain them. But the problem is, just because you hope you never need stockpiles doesn't mean you never will.

The government stockpile consisted of outdated and untested PPE, critical machines that were not in working order, and a woefully inadequate distribution plan. And the actual amount of supplies available was far too small.

So here are a few suggestions:

- Scrap the national stockpile. Instead, every hospital should keep a standard amount of emergency supplies and equipment on-site, based on the number of patients each hospital serves and that hospital's size. This should be mandatory and should be funded via enhanced Medicare payments or a similar mechanism. Having hundreds of stockpiles throughout the country at every major medical facility (and many minor ones) may seem less efficient than having one national stockpile, but it will be more effective, and it will alleviate distribution issues.
- The components and quantities of the stockpile supplies should be determined by a non-partisan panel.
- Each stockpile should be monitored to assure hospital compliance with set standards. Currently, a hospital is required to undergo an outside audit every three years to assure compliance with Medicare rules and regulations. These audits already include surveys of medications and supplies and easily could be expanded to include a survey of emergency stockpiles. If there still is a need for a national stockpile, it also should be audited every three years. Such an audit would have prevented the distribution of thousands of unusable masks and inoperable ventilators.
- The people overseeing the stockpiling – either at hospitals or at a national level – need to be protected from political pressure. Hospitals or states must receive supplies based on their needs and size of the population they serve, not because a local politician is in or out of favor

with a national one.

- Finally, we need to reestablish the CDC as a politically independent, world-leading organization. It must have a clearly defined role in a national disaster or pandemic, and both political parties must accept that role. Accepting or rejecting medical information or advice should not be based on one's party or political ideology. Clearly, I don't think that a president should be the main source of medical information – but neither should other elected officials. In New York City, as Mayor Bill de Blasio told people to go see their physicians if they were sick, the health experts advised people to stay home, contact their physician by phone, and only go to the hospital if they developed significant symptoms. Medical experts need to lead the way in communicating to the public. They should take the lead at regular press conferences, and politicians should support these experts – not the other way around.

A commission formed to plan for future pandemics– and to evaluate what went wrong with our management of Covid-19 – could use these action items as a starting point. Implementing these changes will make a significant difference when the next threat arises.

**On October 2, 2020**

- President Donald Trump and First Lady Melania Trump test positive for Covid-19; DOW stock futures fall more than 400 points in response.
- The city of Rome mandates that all people wear masks outdoors.
- Major League Baseball reports no Covid-19 cases among players for 33 consecutive days.

CHAPTER SEVENTEEN

# Heroes Without Capes

*"Real heroes don't wear capes. Real superheroes wear uniforms and badges and stethoscopes! Real superheroes are members of our military, law enforcement, and first responders."*

**Dean Cain**
Actor, *Lois & Clark: The New Adventures of Superman*
June 2018

The nurses and medical staff at Holy Name all wear different color scrubs. This allows patients, visitors, and staff to more easily identify people from different departments. Navy blue signifies the OR; white scrubs and black pants are medical nurses; all black scrubs are ED physicians; khaki tops and black bottoms are radiology, physical therapy, and lab; and red scrubs signify an outside vendor (pharmaceutical or medical supply representatives).

About a week after our first Covid-19 patients arrived, we designated gray scrubs for those working with Covid-19 patients. Initially, gray scrubs were limited to several specific areas of the hospital. But soon, we were all wearing gray – signifying that we were all in this together. No matter your role at Holy Name before the time of Covid-19, you were now part of our Covid-19 response team. This sea of gray and PPE made us all look alike and, in a way, reflected our common purpose – and, unfortunately, our common mood.

Since it was difficult to tell us apart, staff put large pieces of masking tape on the back of their scrubs and wrote their names (or sometimes a nickname) with a Sharpie. Our scrubs looked almost like sports jerseys, reminding us that we were a team all fighting one opponent: Covid-19.

Utility workers have a similar experience when facing a big storm, working together for tireless, long hours fighting for a common cause. For years (and even decades) after, they will share the memories of battling Superstorm Sandy, Hurricane Katrina, and other massive weather events. Covid-19 was our storm of storms. It pulled us together and will serve as a defining moment for those of us who lived through it.

I cannot understate the bravery of Holy Name's nurses, doctors, medical technicians, patient transporters, cafeteria workers, construction workers, and countless others. They knew they were dealing with something that could infect and kill them, as well as the people they loved, and that we had no known cure. But they reported to work, put in extra hours, and did what needed to be done. They displayed an exceptional level of courage, and that courage deserves recognition.

Ashley Blanchard is a nurse who trained at Holy Name about 15 years ago. She started her career as a medical/surgical nurse, then became our Manager of Infection Control, tasked with leading our fight against infections. During the pandemic, Ashley served as our main liaison to the local and state Departments of Health, traced all of our staff infections, educated staff on donning and doffing, and worked on the team that developed all Covid-19 policies and procedures, in addition to a myriad of other responsibilities.

Throughout the pandemic, it seemed that Ashley never left the hospital. One day, I told her she had to go home, decompress, and get some sleep. She agreed, but a few hours later when I visited the ICU, I found her ducking around a corner, trying to hide from me. This happened with other staff as well. No matter how much I asked them to prioritize their own well-being, they insisted on staying at the hospital to serve their patients.

Suraj worked closely with Ashley to ensure that everyone followed the right procedures to limit infection within the hospital. He is a great communicator. During the pandemic, he and I produced a weekly Holy Name video update that we sent to all hospital staff. These were short video clips about the current state of the hospital: how many Covid-19 patients we had, updates on PPE supplies, where we were with construction of the new Covid-19 wards, and, of course, stories of recovered patients and logistical successes.

Many of our staff have told me that they really appreciated these regular updates – they were a welcomed respite from the endless days of caring for patient after patient. They said that the videos acknowledged their work and helped them feel like they were part of an important team (which they were), pulling together for the good of our patients and the overall community.

Suraj also co-hosts a podcast called "Recommended Daily Dose." He and another member of the medical staff, Dr. Clenton Coleman, discuss various medical topics in both a humorous and informative way. They have dealt extensively with Covid-19 on their podcast, but some other interesting segments include *Mosquitos Suck, Dr. Google Will See You Now*, and *You'll Go Blind!! and Other Medical Myths Debunked.* If you like podcasts, give it a try.

* * * * *

Staff members were extremely flexible about pitching in whenever and wherever needed. Many staff members assumed new roles during Covid-19. At one daily meeting, Dawn Mattera, who ran our ICU, reported, "We're okay on our ventilator supply for the next 12 hours or so, but we don't have enough critical care nurses."

Donna Vaglio, our OR director, spoke up. "Since we don't have any elective surgeries, we have nurses from the OR and PACU" – the post-anesthesia care unit – "who could move down to the ICU. They would need to initially be paired with critical care nurses, but would the extra hands help?" Within hours, the reinforcements from the OR and PACU arrived in the ICU.

Throughout the pandemic, the ICU was the most challenging and emotionally draining place for our staff. The physicians did an amazing job rounding from patient to patient, evaluating each one and making necessary medication or ventilator adjustments, but it was the nurses who spent hours and, in many cases, days and weeks with our ICU patients. These were not typical ICU patients. Many of them were relatively young, and unfortunately, many of them died. Because family could not be present, the nurses filled in. They held patients' hands, they spoke reassuring words, and they cried a lot.

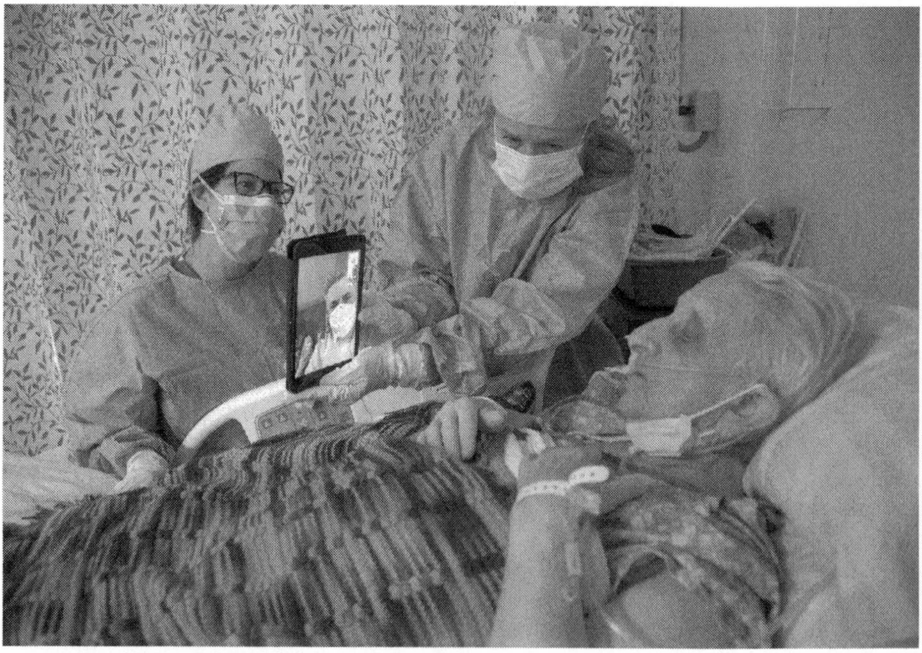

Nursing in the ICU is always challenging, but the challenges of Covid-19 would have been unimaginable just a few months before the pandemic started.

Some doctors also took on new roles. One day, Dr. Luke Eyerman came into my office, plopped himself down across from me, and asked, "What can I do to help?"

Luke, a terrific young primary care physician, was feeling underutilized since many of his patients were cancelling appointments. I thought for a second. The critical care physicians were beginning to get overwhelmed by the extraordinary number of Covid-19 patients, and some of the older primary care physicians, or those who had underlying medical conditions, were understandably reluctant to treat Covid-19 patients.

"Luke, could you cover the non-critical Covid-19 patients? You would stay in regular communication with the critical care physicians in case patients get worse, but we just don't have enough doctors seeing Covid-19 patients right now."

Luke nodded enthusiastically. "Absolutely."

A week later, Luke not only was doing rounds in the Covid-19 wards but had recruited five other primary care physicians to join him.

The whole staff stepped it up, not just the nurses and doctors. Allison Sinclair usually helped to manage our physician network (a 250 physician multi-specialty group that works directly for Holy Name), but during Covid-19, she ran our telemedicine program. Allison recruited nurse practitioners from around our network to call and stay in touch with all of our suspected and confirmed patients with cases of Covid-19.

We took care of more than 7,000 patients via telemedicine – checking temperatures and oxygen levels, assessing the need for hospitalization, and answering questions. This program was not just key to patient health, but also kept patients out of the ED unless absolutely necessary – which was crucial in keeping our ED volume as manageable as possible. Telemedicine played a small role in patient care prior to the pandemic, but I suspect that once we are through Covid-19, it will be key to making sure our patients continue to receive the best care possible.

It was not just Holy Name staff who stepped up during the pandemic. Governor Murphy put out a call for assistance to medical workers from around the country to come to New Jersey. My nephew Zach was among those who responded.

Zach, a nurse anesthetist, worked at an upstate New York hospital that had not yet been impacted by the pandemic. He had previously worked as a critical care nurse in a neurological ICU. In March, he and his fiancée were sick. The timing and the symptoms were right for Covid-19, but testing was not yet available. Zach was convinced that they both had Covid-19, and I assumed he was right. They quarantined and then resumed their lives, confident that they had some form of immunity, and one less thing to worry about.

Zach had exactly the training and experience we needed at Holy Name. When I called him and suggested he come help us and our patients, he expressed some reservations. But although he was a bit anxious about working in a Covid-19 unit, he thought he was immune and knew he could help – so he agreed.

Zach traveled to Holy Name three times (each time for three days). He worked in our Covid-19 ICU alongside our nurses and critical care physicians, assisting with ventilator management. He weaned patients off ventilators, he placed central lines, and he assisted in code blues. Most importantly, he allowed our staff to get some much-needed rest.

On the last morning of his third visit, Zach pulled me aside when we passed in the hallway. He told me that he had had a restless night and hadn't gotten much sleep. He was exhausted and glad to be heading home, but on his drive that night, he developed a fever.

The next morning, he called out sick for his shift at his hospital. He went for a Covid-19 test and self-quarantined as he awaited the result. His symptoms worsened, and several days later he and his fiancée both received positive Covid-

9 test results. Apparently, their earlier bout of sickness had not been Covid-19.

They both worsened, with symptoms of extreme fatigue, fever, cough, nd shortness of breath. I felt terribly guilty. I didn't know for sure how Zach got nfected, but it seemed likely that it had happened at Holy Name, and I was sure hat he had spread his infection to his fiancée.

When he was well enough for us to speak, I asked him if he had any houghts about how he got infected. He told me that he couldn't be sure, but that e remembered a specific incident when he was so close to a patient's mouth hat, despite wearing an N-95 mask covered by a surgical mask, he sensed he night be inhaling the patient's breath. It wasn't pleasant, he said, but as a nurse nesthetist, it was something he had experienced before. At the time, he had uickly dismissed it. Was it because he assumed he was immune? Or was it ecause he was willing to put himself at risk to help his patients? At that point it o longer mattered, and I was just relieved that he was getting better.

Thankfully, both Zach and his fiancée fully recovered, and they are both ack to work. In fact, Zach continues to work at Holy Name when he is able to, nd he has become a valuable member of our team.

I was concerned that many of our staff would get infected like Zach did. Of course, I didn't want them to get sick, but selfishly, I was also concerned that f a significant number of them were not able to work, we wouldn't be able to ake care of our patients. Aside from ensuring that the staff was as protected as ossible and attempting to recruit additional staff, I did not have a good solution.

I remember one day running into Dr. Harris Tesher, one of the critical care physicians, in the hallway. He told me that Dr. Richard May, another critical care physician, had gone home with a fever. My heart sank. I thought, *This is the beginning. The staff is going to be decimated.*

Harris must have seen the look on my face, but he smiled and said, "I can't believe how happy I am that one of my colleagues has the flu." Richard had had a fever and fatigue, so he was tested for Covid-19, dreading the worst. Everyone was relieved when his swab came back positive only for influenza A. He was back to work in five days.

At Holy Name, only two ED physicians and one infectious disease physician developed Covid-19; they all recovered uneventfully. Remarkably, none of the critical care physicians, the doctors working most closely with Covid-19 patients, or the critical care nurses became infected – a testament to how effective negative pressure rooms and proper PPE can be in preventing infections.

* * * * *

I cannot even begin to capture the range of emotions and personal tragedies that our staff dealt with during this first wave of Covid-19. Each day as they came to work, they were anxious, knowing that their patients may have worsened, or even died, during the night. Too often, this stress exacerbated the heartbreak of losing their own loved ones. Some of our staff lost neighbors, friends, husbands, uncles, aunts, and in-laws to Covid-19.

In addition to caring for their patients, two nurses, Eniko Szecsi and Isabel Pena (whose son, Xavier, is also a Holy Name employee), regularly checked up on their husbands, Istvan and Santiago, who both were battling Covid-19 at Holy Name. When it became clear that further aggressive treatment was going to be of no benefit, Eniko and Isabel decided to withdraw care and allow their husbands to have peaceful deaths. Istvan and Santiago were transferred out of the ICU, given medicines to make them comfortable, and then taken off ventilators. They died peacefully, two days apart from one another.

Eniko, Isabel, and Xavier suffered a horrible loss, but because of their ositions at the hospital, they were able to be present for Istvan and Santiago's inal days – a small but meaningful comfort. Neither nurse missed a scheduled hift, even though we told them to take as much time as they wanted – they knew heir patients needed them.

We also lost staff.

Two of the first Holy Name employees to die from Covid-19 were not linical staff, but were just as crucial to the running of the hospital. They were ixtures in the organization. Everyone knew them, and their loss had a remendous impact on the entire staff.

Andres Benitez was one of the first people I met when I joined Holy Name. He was a food service worker who had worked at Holy Name for more han 15 years before he fell ill. I saw him regularly in the cafeteria at lunchtime, nd he always had a smile and a funny story to share. He lightened the mood of veryone he talked to.

In early March, Andres missed several days of work with mild Covid-19 ymptoms. He came to our ED as his symptoms worsened and was tested for ikely viral causes. These results all came back negative, so we also tested him or Covid-19. Five days later, those results came back positive. Andres was ospitalized for more than two weeks. He died in our ICU.

Word of his death spread quickly, accompanied by a deep grief. A nember of our team had been taken by this horrible disease. It drove home the isk we were all taking every day. Many of us felt a sense of despair; I know I lid. Andres's brother was also a Covid-19 patient at the hospital at the time. Vhen we informed him of his brother's death, he was fighting for his own life, lone, separated from his family. He eventually recovered.

The next morning, we held a service in the hospital kitchen with

Andres's fellow food service workers. At the end of the service, we had a brief moment of silence in his honor, heads bowed. When I looked up, I scanned the room. In the faces of his co-workers, I not only saw sadness, but fear. I realized that I likely had the same expression on my face. We were all wondering, could one of us be next? But as hard as it was, we reluctantly moved on. I spent a lot of time that day thinking about my mother's words when our neighbor had died fifty years earlier: take the time you need, then rejoin the world. We had work to do.

* * * * *

One time when Jesus Villaluz won a 50/50 raffle at a Holy Name fundraiser, he shared it with his fellow patient transporters. It was the kind of generous action that endeared him to his co-workers.

Jesus rarely called out sick during his 27 years with Holy Name, but he didn't come into work when he developed symptoms consistent with Covid-19. Over the next few days, he worsened and made plans to come to the hospital for a Covid-19 test. Before he could, his breathing became so labored that he called for an ambulance. When he arrived at the hospital, he had already been placed on a ventilator by the ambulance team. His Covid-19 test came back positive two days after his admission, though we had already assumed that he had the virus because of his symptoms. Despite our best efforts, he continued to worsen. Jesus died just 10 days after Andres. His death left the hospital numb.

Shortly after his death, staff members gathered in two lines outside of the ICU, everyone in masks. After a moment of silence, Dave Van Bever pushed the bed carrying Jesus's body, covered by a white sheet, down the corridor. Staff reached out to touch the stretcher. Some who knew Jesus well reached out to touch his arm beneath the sheet.

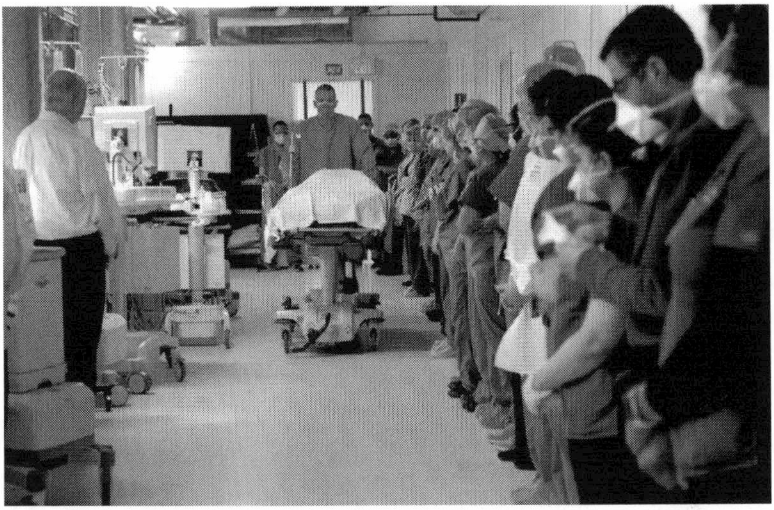

Staff bidding goodbye to one of our own.

Throughout the pandemic, we tried to have some light moments. The staff would gather, typically around food, and would talk about better days, family members, and planned vacations, and even make some jokes. For a few days after Jesus died, this stopped. It was hard to find even brief moments of joy after the loss of someone who was such an integral part of Holy Name.

Sadly, these were not the only members of the Holy Name team that we lost to Covid-19. This pandemic has devastated healthcare workers around the globe, and every colleague lost is sorely missed. Their deaths leave a hole in the quilt of our community.

**Covid-19 Healthcare Worker Deaths**
**As of September 3, 2020**
Source: Amnesty International

| | |
|---|---|
| • Worldwide Total | >7,000 |
| • Mexico | 1,320 |
| • United States | 1,077 |
| • Brazil | 634 |

CHAPTER EIGHTEEN

# Insights

*"But as sure as spring comes to the forest, incidental beauty emerges from crisis. This is also human nature. We can't help but hope for good things. Hope for survival, for better medicine, for widespread testing, for more ventilators, for intuitive leadership, for a successful vaccine. Hope for the day we will gather to grieve what's gone and celebrate being together again."*

**Mary Pembleton**
Writer
"A Pulse of Joy Amid Tragedy," *New York Times*
April 20, 2020

The alarm goes off at 4:45 a.m. I'm tempted for a few brief seconds to hit the snooze button, as I am every morning, but I remind myself that I will feel the same way when the alarm goes off again in 15 minutes. I don't want to disturb Eileen, so I keep the lights off as I move to the bathroom, amazed, as always, at how unsteady I feel on my feet for the first few minutes after I get out of bed. I think about how I never felt unsteady like this when I was 30.

I laid out my running attire the night before, which now includes a mask, and by 5 a.m., I am out the door with headphones in place, listening to "This American Life." I head down the elevator from my 13th floor New York City apartment. The building is silent, too early even for the doorman. The streets are quiet as I start my four-mile run, working my way toward the bike path on the West Side. I pass a sleeping homeless person just past the overpass that gets me to the path, and I head north.

I was never a great runner, even in my physical "prime." At 57, I'm now hunched over with arthritic hips. I'm slow, but still steady.

About three miles in, I pass the workout equipment on the running path, a pull-up bar, a captain's chair, and a bench dip, and pause to do my three sets of 10 pull-ups. I struggle, but I mostly get it done. I work my way back to the apartment aerobically strong, but my hips really feel it. Eileen frequently tells me that I shouldn't be running so much, but it's one of the few things that clears my mind in the midst of this pandemic, so I persevere.

A key lesson I learned during this pandemic is to start by taking care of yourself. We all – the frontline workers, those who got Covid-19, those who sheltered in place and felt isolated and lonely, those who lost jobs, brides- and grooms-to-be who postponed weddings, and really everyone in our society – suffered during the pandemic. It is critical that we focus on getting ourselves through this as healthily as possible – physically and emotionally. That's why, almost every day, I make time to run.

After focusing on ourselves, we must focus on our colleagues. As I walked through a ward one day in the middle of the pandemic, as usual, I thanked each member of the staff, trying to stay as positive as possible. While some days were harder than others, the staff's attitudes in the midst of the worst medical crisis they had ever seen – or likely would ever see again – were incredible. It struck me that day, and in subsequent days, that the staff was enthusiastically thanking me back.

They were on the frontline, much more than I was, and, frankly, I was less deserving of thanks. Then I realized: they had been seeing reports on the news of other hospitals without enough PPE, and they were truly grateful for the efforts that Holy Name had taken to ensure their safety. They appreciated both the precautions to protect them, and the little things – such as the Zen Den, free food, dry cleaning, and haircuts.

As the pandemic progressed and the scientific debate raged over the airborne spread of Covid-19, I appreciated even more what Steve and his team had accomplished with negative pressure rooms. Although reasonable scientists can differ on their views of airborne spread, if there is any possibility that a virus spreads in this manner, why wouldn't healthcare facilities make the necessary, relatively small investment to protect their staff? As hospitals prepare for the next wave, or even the next pandemic, they should develop plans to create negative pressure rooms quickly and efficiently. And when building new hospitals or new wings in old hospitals, medical organizations should build the capability for additional negative pressure rooms into the initial construction.

A hospital can have fancy, expensive equipment and new, shiny rooms, but the care given and received is only as good as a hospital's frontline staff. When they feel appreciated and safe, they provide better care. It's our responsibility as their employer to ensure they know that their work is valued and that we are doing everything we can to keep them out of harm's way – especially in a time of crisis. It's just the right thing to do.

* * * * *

During my residency, one of my mentors told me, "In most situations, you should not be an early adopter of new medicines or new techniques." He illustrated his point: "If someone developed a vaccine for the common cold, take the vaccine, but don't be the first one to take it. It's okay to wait awhile."

This makes clinical sense. When the FDA initially approves new treatments, these treatments are still being formally studied for safety in what is called "phase four" or "post-marketing" trials.

We really do not know how truly safe new medications are until they have been in the market for a period of time. For example, numerous blood pressure medications have completed post marketing studies. We know that they are safe and effective, so is there a need to try a new blood pressure medication hat has just hit the market and doesn't have the same proven safety profile? The imple answer is, almost always, no.

Numerous medications have been removed from the market for safety ssues after they were initially released. For example, two drugs, Rofecoxib, a on-steroidal anti-inflammatory medication used primarily to treat arthritis, and ibutramine, an appetite suppressant, were removed from the market after being hown to significantly increase the risk of heart attacks and strokes. If a nanufacturer claims that a new drug is better, cheaper, or easier to administer, ou can almost always afford to wait and see if the claims hold true.

So, "It's okay to wait awhile" makes sense. However, my lesson from Covid-19 (building on my experience with HIV/AIDS) is that this rule has xceptions. Potentially life-threatening diseases without known treatments equire innovation, creativity, and sometimes an abandonment of the level of aution we are often comfortable with. If you were dying of HIV/AIDS in the 980s, it made sense to try new experimental drugs. In my view, treatments for Covid-19 also meet these criteria, as might certain preventative treatments such s a Covid-19 vaccine.

* * * * *

In a crisis, it's important to step back, pause, and exercise common ense. This is important advice even when we are not in the midst of a crisis, but often it unfortunately falls by the wayside.

I had a call from a friend, Tim, at the beginning of the pandemic. His dult son, Calvin, had just moved out of his apartment in New York City and was back home after eight years. Calvin had asthma and they were concerned that he night be prone to a more severe case of Covid-19 (the scientific evidence on this s still mixed).

They were ahead of the curve in taking many precautions; Calvin left the city several weeks ahead of many of his peers, for instance. After discussing whether Calvin's girlfriend could visit (not ideal if she was traveling back and forth from her parents' home) and laying out some additional precautions (staying away from people outside of their immediate family), Tim seemed comfortable with a plan that would minimize Calvin's risk of contracting the virus.

However, when I checked back in with Tim a few days later, he mentioned that he and his son had gone to the grocery store to stock up for a few weeks. I couldn't keep myself from saying, a little sternly, "Tim, why did you *both* go to the store? The whole point of our conversation the other day was to protect Calvin as much as possible. There's no reason he should be going to the store when he's living at home with you."

Dealing with a pandemic – one that might linger with us for a while (and potentially kill us or our loved ones) – means learning what the risks are, acknowledging the risks, and taking common sense actions to reduce those risks as much as possible, hopefully in ways that have as small a negative impact on our lives as possible. Wearing masks, washing hands, avoiding crowds, and, yes, having just one family member make grocery runs (during off-hours if possible) may be a nuisance, but these are actions that make sense and significantly reduce our risk of getting infected.

We need to be persistent in taking simple but effective precautions. For example, wearing a mask is a small price to pay to protect ourselves, our loved ones, and our communities.

Another lesson learned during Covid-19 is that sometimes, we need to consciously stop and rethink our actions and reactions. This requires some effort on our part, and we need to be willing to buck social norms. Very early on in the pandemic, Eileen began to share my experiences at the hospital and what I was learning about the virus with friends and family. Things happened so quickly that she sent texts nearly every day. One day, I told Eileen to communicate that the situation had become very serious and that our friends and family should not travel anywhere. Some had trips already booked and questioned whether they really had to cancel their plans. The answer was yes.

A couple of weeks later, Eileen was on the phone with one of her college roommates, Diane, who had received all of Eileen's texts about the virus. Diane, who lives outside of Boston, mentioned that she had just returned from a family funeral in New York. When Eileen asked her why she went – especially since I had advised everyone to stay home – Diane responded, "It was a funeral. How could I not go?"

Of course, our natural reaction to the death of a family member, friend, or co-worker is to go to the funeral to offer our condolences, pay our respects, and say our goodbyes. But during this critical time when community spread had taken hold, it did not make sense in terms of minimizing risk. Funerals were significant spreader events of Covid-19 within communities.

Funeral attendees also spread Covid-19 to their own communities as they traveled back to their hometowns. There are several documented cases of people attending a funeral during the pandemic (for both Covid-19 and non-Covid 19 deaths), becoming infected with Covid-19, and spreading it to another family member who died. The grief of the first funeral was now compounded by a second funeral.

Some of the decisions the pandemic forced us to make were heart wrenching, or left us wringing our hands. Others were mere inconveniences. It is difficult to forego celebrating holidays with family or to miss an important family event such as the birth of a baby or the death of a parent. However, the reality of

Covid-19 requires us all to think differently. Yes, family members or friends may be upset with you for missing an important event. But, although it may seem counterintuitive, the best way to show your concern for both those who die and those who remain is to do so remotely.

Covid-19 changed the way we all live. Eileen and I made changes in our lives, too. At the beginning of the crisis, when we knew so little about the virus, Eileen and I tried hard to keep six feet away from each other. There were no welcome home hugs, she ate dinner at the table while I ate at the couch (which was where I also slept), and we watched the news from different sides of the room instead of side-by-side. She even moved her toothbrush away from mine (I'm not sure if she knew that I noticed that).

When I arrived home each evening, she insisted that I remove my clothes as soon as I entered the apartment, and then go right into the shower. Normally after work, I would make dinner for us both. I love to cook and find it relaxing, but Eileen wouldn't let me in the kitchen – she didn't want me to touch anything just in case I was infected.

Eileen was particularly worried about this because her sister, Suzanne, was receiving treatment at Holy Name for cancer, and Eileen had been visiting her every day. This was at the very start of the pandemic before we had banned all visitations at the hospital. As our number of Covid-19 patients increased, I told Eileen that I thought she should stop visiting Suzanne because of my increased exposure. It was too risky for her to be around her sister. Suzanne's doctors began checking in on her from the hallway in case they, too, had been exposed and were infected. While we were all relieved when Suzanne was finally discharged, Eileen's plan to go home with her to help with her recovery was not possible.

But despite the inconveniences, the pandemic reminded us of a time when our lives were simpler. On the weekends, we walked to a nearby park, bringing along a blanket, a board game, and some wine and cheese. When I was a medical student in Washington, D.C., this was often how we spent our weekends.

We also took long walks in Manhattan, something we had done when we first moved to New York City decades earlier. Living on the salaries of a medical resident and a starting teacher, we hadn't had much money to see movies or theater. So we spent our free time exploring the city, broke, but happy.

We had relished these long walks, especially on quiet Sunday mornings. We enjoyed window shopping for things we could not afford, people watching as we strolled through the street fairs, and trying foods from street vendors. We loved theater, but rarely could afford Broadway. Instead, the people on the streets were our entertainment – a native wind instrument troop from El Salvador, break dancers, a landscape painter, and scores of ordinary people walking by.

Eileen and I had loved the city when we lived there in the late 1980s and early 1990s, despite our lack of funds. That's why, after our kids all moved out of the house, we moved from the suburbs of Northern New Jersey back to New York.

When we go on our walks now, we still enjoy watching the diverse and interesting people who we pass. We don't stop in restaurants or sample street fair food, but our walks today are just as peaceful as they were thirty years ago.

I am not alone in finding connections in the time of Covid-19. We have friends like Tim, who have really valued having their adult children move back home, or others who have made a point to call elderly relatives more often and, as a result, have built stronger relationships with them.

The Covid-19 pandemic will be a time many will look back on with frustration and sadness. However, there will be many who look back on it with mixed emotions, as a time when they reconnected with their parents or children, interacted more with their siblings, read more books (or even wrote one), took up a new hobby like painting or knitting, spent time creating a garden, or simply focused on the simple things that a family can do together.

The Covid-19 pandemic has certainly been a time of great hardships – not just for those that lost loved ones or those who suffered long recoveries, but for those that suffered economically as well, with lost jobs, evictions, or the uncertainty of how they might be able to feed their family. The country failed to come together to help those most negatively affected by Covid-19, something for which I believe future generation will – and should – judge us harshly.

However, for me, spending quiet, simple time with Eileen has been a pleasure. She has even let me back in the kitchen, where I spend most of my weekends trying new recipes. Against the backdrop of Covid-19, we need to celebrate these small silver linings.

**On October 28, 2020**

- 2.8 million cases and 40,000 new deaths in the preceding week worldwide.
- 8.7 million cases and 226,773 deaths in the U.S total.
- France imposes a new national lockdown as Covid-19 cases rise.
- Dodgers and Lakers fans are asked to quarantine in Los Angeles following championship wins and outbreaks of cases after celebration parties.

CHAPTER NINETEEN

# Forging Ahead

*"We're going to have many more hospitalizations, and that will inevitably lead to more deaths. So, this is an untenable situation."*

**Dr. Anthony Fauci**
Director, National Institute of Allergy and Infectious Diseases
October 28, 2020

The restaurants of New Jersey reopened (outdoors, with limited indoor eating), as did the parks and the Jersey Shore. On the boardwalk, most people wore masks, and on the beach, people sat a little further from each other. You could go to the water's edge and watch the never-ending waves lapping at the golden sands, and it almost seemed as if we were not in the middle of a pandemic. But, as of November 2020, we still don't know how long this pandemic will last.

After the first Covid-19 wave in New Jersey crested and the threat began to diminish, I tuned in to a Zoom panel held by *The Record*, the daily newspaper in Bergen County. At one point, Lindy Washburn, a health reporter for the paper, commented, "We had a failure of imagination – we just didn't think it could get this bad." Lindy used the past tense, but I am still concerned. As I write this, we are at the start of the dreaded second wave, and I fear that we again are unable to imagine what might be coming.

How bad will this wave be? That will depend on many factors: possible viral genetic mutations, people continuing to socially distance and wear masks, government action on shutting down businesses (locally or more widely), the effectiveness and availability of a vaccine, and the willingness of people to take it. Despite our best efforts, this virus could still win the battle.

People around the world are wondering what the days and months ahead will look like. At Holy Name, we are certainly better prepared for the coming months than we were in March. We have our own stockpile of PPE and ventilators, and all the negative pressure rooms that we built are still in place. We have somewhat better therapeutics. Our staff has a better understanding of this disease and how to combat it. As I walk the halls of the hospital, spirits are upbeat, but we should not underestimate the stress and strain this pandemic has had on healthcare workers. What they went through in March and April was inconceivable, and we're about to ask them to do it again.

Just as Drs. McCormack and Pitkin and Mother Brown planned for this pandemic a hundred years ago by founding Holy Name, we need to make sure that we are diligent in preparing for the future. Hospitals, however, play only a partial role in this task. Historically, hospitals and the entire U.S. healthcare system, for good or bad, have been better at responding to illness than preventing it – but this needs to change. So, what actions do we need to take?

Individuals must entertain and be prepared for the possibility that the worst is yet to come. It is worth repeating – wear masks, wash hands, socially distance, and self-quarantine if you think you might have been exposed. These are the same actions taken 100 years ago to ward off the Spanish flu. They are still relevant today because they work.

Recently, I watched a *60 Minutes* interview with Dr. Christina Brennan, the Vice President of Clinical Research at Northwell Health. When asked, "If you had to choose between a mask or a vaccine, what would you choose?" she responded without hesitation: "Masks are more important." She's right. Masks are our most effective weapon. Even when we have a safe and effective vaccine, ve must continue to wear masks until the vaccine is widely available and taken y a significant portion of the world's population.

Wearing masks is crucial to decrease the impact of the second wave. ndividuals cannot stop wearing masks even after getting a negative test result. Remember, Covid-19 tests are just not that good, and we must understand the eality of imperfect testing. As we can now test many more people, we will see nore false negative results – so continue to be cautious, even if your test comes back negative.

And get a flu shot this year and every year, because we don't know when he next Covid-19 or the next Spanish flu is coming. Except for exceedingly rare ircumstances, the flu shot is safe. The benefits of getting a flu shot, both for you personally and for the nation, greatly outweigh the potential risks. If you are not villing to do it for yourself, do it for the ones you love.

Every year, we have a hospital-wide initiative to make sure that all of our mployees get their flu shots. This year, the State of New Jersey mandated that ll healthcare workers receive a flu shot, with very limited exceptions. This hould become standard practice for the nation's healthcare workers.

Flu season is always a challenging time for healthcare facilities. Based on the severity of the flu season, the challenges can be mild to overwhelming. Flu always causes a significant increase in hospital admissions, which can in turn back up our ED, decrease the efficient operation of all areas of the hospital, and ultimately affect the quality of care we provide. Although flu does not bring all of the challenges of Covid-19, it still is a highly infectious disease that kills vulnerable people every year.

Flu and Covid-19 have similar symptoms, which creates a challenge when trying to diagnose, treat, and prevent infections. The flu season of 2020-2021 will be unlike any other we have faced, and until we have minimized the impact of Covid-19, this may become our new normal. As one of my fellow administrators put it, "Dealing with Covid-19 was a challenge, but we were able to focus on just Covid-19 patients. It's actually harder to be back in a world with both infectious Covid-19 patients and non-Covid-19 patients – and on top of that we could have a really bad flu season." She couldn't have been more on target – we need to be prepared for Covid-19, flu, and other infectious diseases, and at th same time provide high-quality care for non-infectious patients (those with strokes, heart attacks, appendectomies, etc.). Again, we have to look at our workflows and processes to be sure we can keep all of our patients and staff safe, focusing on the separation of infectious patients from non-infectious patients.

Unlike Ebola and SARS, which created a false sense of security because they did not have a significant impact on the U.S. population or its healthcare system, this pandemic has made Holy Name better prepared for this flu season (and future ones), as well as for additional waves of Covid-19 or whatever other disease may come next. We need to maintain and build on this preparedness and make sure we do not slip backwards.

* * * * *

During the pandemic, I tried to immediately alert the staff whenever a problem arose, and to share my proposed solution (if I had one). To be frank, these were not always solutions I loved. However, I told the team not to reject a proposed solution unless they could offer a better one. We would then brainstorm the problem and potential solutions, almost always finding a better option than the one I had started with. These solutions were often unorthodox, but I was proud to have developed a leadership style that encouraged creative thinking and problem-solving.

Innovation and outside-the-box thinking will be critical to getting us through future waves of Covid-19, or the next healthcare crisis. Some healthcare nd government leaders will possess this creativity themselves, but others will oster an environment that encourages and nurtures innovation by others. Lives vere, and will continue to be, saved by transforming our ordinary processes and ystems in extraordinary ways. In the highly regulated and bureaucratic ealthcare world we live in today, transformation sometimes requires a villingness to bend or break the rules, and leaders to give the go ahead to do so.

Leaders can deal with rules in three ways:

- A **good leader** knows the rules, understands the implications of breaking them, and breaks them when the rewards outweigh the risks.
- A **mediocre leader** understands the rules and sticks to them no matter the consequences.
- A **bad leader** either doesn't take the time to learn the rules or breaks the rules without considering the implications or risks.

The best leaders surround themselves with people who will say, "Let's discuss this before you break the rules," and create environments that encourage others to challenge them in this way.

During Covid-19, the need to break certain rules was blatantly obvious and, to some degree, sanctioned. The Governor of New Jersey declared a state of emergency, allowing us to make decisions that may have broken the rules in some cases, but that also allowed us to better protect our staff and care for patients. Should we reuse masks or treat them with UV light? Should we import non-FDA-approved tests from Germany? Should we develop and use an "unapproved" piece of equipment (the ISO-pod) that will decrease the spread of the virus?

For me, rule breaking is almost inevitable in times of crisis, but if we are going to head off these crises and be better prepared for the next one, we must also encourage beyond-the-rules thinking in non-crisis times.

Sometimes, healthcare leaders must accept the risks of breaking the rules for the good of the patients and staff they serve. And remarkably, sometimes when the dust settles, this process ultimately changes the rules.

* * * * *

Friends, family, and even the media frequently ask me about the state of our current Covid-19 therapeutics. "Are patients doing better because we have better treatments?" "Is the worst behind us?" "What happens next?" I am concerned that there is a misperception that the few small breakthroughs scientists have had will dramatically change the mortality rate in the second or future waves. I do believe that regular use of remdesivir and dexamethasone to treat Covid-19 has had a very small impact. I am somewhat more optimistic about the potential benefits of monoclonal antibodies. However, this treatment is expensive and is not going to be widely available. As of early October, the U.S. had purchased 300,000 doses, but only 50,000 of them had been produced. This is woefully inadequate; if this medicine is the answer, demand will quickly outstrip supply, not unlike the demand for testing in the early days of the pandemic.

Sadly, I believe with our current available treatments, we are on a path to lose another 250,000 Americans before we get through this horrible pandemic.

* * * * *

As of today, we do not know if an initial Covid-19 infection will provide immunity against future infections, make patients more vulnerable to future infections, or have no impact on future infections. The Spanish flu disproportionately affected young adults, perhaps because their exposure to a different, earlier flu may have caused the antibodies of these individuals to react oo strongly, hyper-inflaming and often killing them. Older patients who had een infected with a different flu earlier in their lives may have developed a ross-immunity to Spanish flu, which might have protected them. We just don't now how our bodies will react to Covid-19, but the medical community needs to e prepared for the possibility that this pandemic may affect our patients for ears or decades to come.

At the time of publication, we have received preliminary data that two Covid-19 vaccine candidates are 90-95 percent effective, but until we have final lata reviewed by the FDA these positive preliminary results are just that: preliminary. It is likely that these results will be confirmed, but even if the vaccines are found to be effective and safe, they will have minimal impact over he next few months. We will then need to face the challenges of distribution and convincing all people to be vaccinated. It is likely that the remarkable vaccine levelopment story of Covid-19 will end this pandemic, but will we eventually radicate Covid-19? I doubt it. In all likelihood, patients and healthcare workers vill add Covid-19 to the list of infectious diseases that we battle on a regular basis, and its variants, mutations, and long-term effects will be around for some ime. We need to open our minds to these possibilities and adjust our public policy accordingly.

So, how will healthcare change post-Covid-19?

My inner optimist imagines a future where we develop a safe and effective vaccine, and therapeutics that will allow us to return to normal. A future vhere we learn from our mistakes and are better prepared for what inevitably vill come next, where we build on the new level of cooperation between neighboring healthcare facilities and reestablish the U.S. and the CDC as world leaders in developing and promoting science-based health policy.

The realist in me knows that some of this will be hard to achieve, especially in our current hyper-politicized environment. A vaccine will not eradicate the disease. I expect that we will continue to see some level of Covid-19 for years to come, with intermittent outbreaks that will require localized responses, including closing down restaurants, schools, or even cities or states. If we need to take a Covid-19 vaccine every year or two, like the flu shot, it is even more unlikely that the virus will disappear.

I am also concerned that the politicization of Covid-19 will hinder widespread vaccinations. As a country, we must realize that the key to economic recovery is, first and foremost, a medical solution. People will resume their normal routines when they feel safe.

Let me end with one last story.

Sister Patricia Lynch, Holy Name's CEO before Mike, who, on her deathbed, told him to take care of her hospital, had an enormous adornment attached to the front of Holy Name. Looking at it, one might think it's a cross, but it isn't; she did not want to feature a Catholic symbol that might make people of other faiths feel unwelcome. She instead chose an ankh, a symbol from ancient Egypt that represents life. An ankh has a circle at the top, a horizontal line across its middle that resembles arms, and sweeping lines down and out that resemble a skirt.

While the ankh has adorned Holy Name's facade since 1992, Steve enhanced the ankh in remembrance of those we lost to Covid-19. Inside the circle, he placed red lights in the shape of a heart, one for each patient who died of Covid-19 at Holy Name. He surrounded the entire ankh with 7,000 white lights, representing the patients treated successfully at Holy Name during the first wave of Covid-19.

Holy Name sits on a hill and, as you pass it, the ankh shines as a beacon. It is, and will continue to be, a lasting tribute to our patients – those who survived nd those who died – and the hardworking people who cared for them.

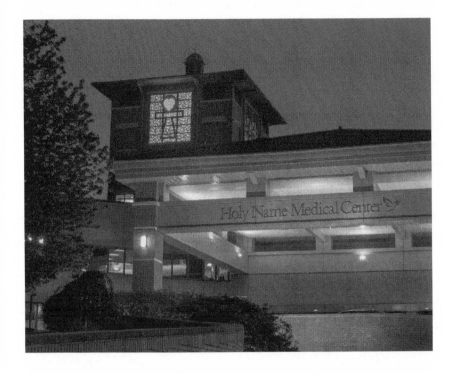

# DEDICATION

This book is dedicated to all those who died from Covid-19. Particularly, those members of the Holy Name community:

**Jesus Villaluz**

**Andres Benitez**

**Severiana Gimenez**

**Murray Hamada**

**Istvan Szecsi**

**Santiago De La Cruz**

**Robert Hurley**

**Enid Acito**

## Acknowledgements

We would first and foremost like to thank our wives, Eileen Jarrett and Betsy Golden, who were editors, idea shapers, and overall supporters of this project. A very special thanks also goes to Dylan Jarrett and Alex Herter for their long hours and efforts on crucial edits and re-writes.

We truly appreciate the friends and family who read, edited, and made suggestions on drafts, specifically Stefi Jarrett, Randi Kestenbaum, Jacqueline Schimmel, Pon Chellaraj, Annalise Roberts, Kathleen Fitzgerald, Melissa Ficuciello, Ed Silver, Mandy Rosengren, and Danica Rosengren. And from Holy Name, thanks for the words of wisdom and help with early drafts: Mike Maron, Ed Ruzinsky, Bob Sommer, Ron White, Randy Tartacoff, Tom Birch, and Ravit Barkama.

A special thanks to three Holy Name colleagues: Jeff Rhode's great photographs both on the covers and in the book helped us tell our story; Michele Acito, for her words of encouragement early on and her willingness to share her memories and experiences of the pandemic; and Emma Yamada, for help with much of the Holy Name data.

Thank you to Jaime Jarrett, Petra Jarrett, and Casey Rosengren for being there for us during the writing of this book and always.

A large shout-out goes to all the phenomenal staff at Holy Name Medical Center, named and unnamed. We apologize for any heroic efforts overlooked. You make a difference every day in the lives that you touch.

About the Authors

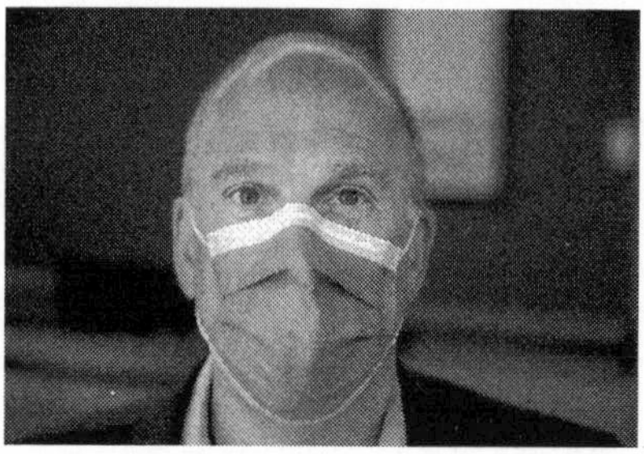

**Dr. Adam Jarrett** – Adam Jarrett, MD, MS is an internal medicine/primary care physician who attended medical school at George Washington University and then completed his residency at New York Hospital Cornell University Medical School. He then went on to the private practice of medicine in Ridgewood and Midland Park, New Jersey as a partner at Prospect Medical Offices. He completed his Master of Science at the Robert F. Wagner Graduate School of Public Service, New York University and then served as Chief Medical Officer at Claxton-Hepburn Medical Center in Ogdensburg, New York. He currently is the Executive Vice President and Chief Medical Officer of Holy Name Medical Center in Teaneck, New Jersey. Dr. Jarrett is a regular medical contributor for national and local broadcast networks and print media, providing commentary on medical topics and public health policy, in addition to sharing insights on the Covid-19 pandemic.

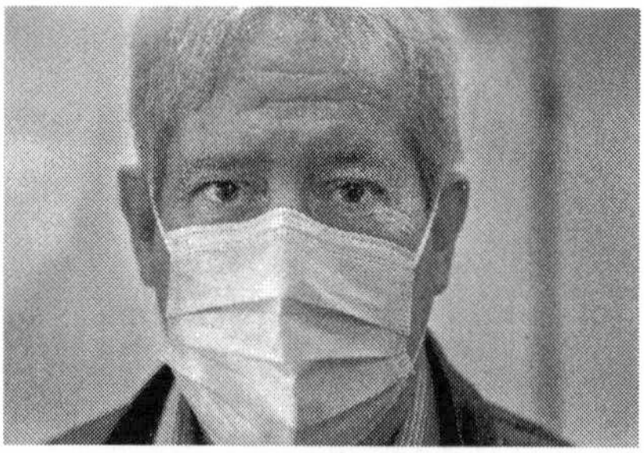

**Paul Rosengren** – Paul Rosengren is an internal and external communications professional. He has been the speechwriter for the Presidents/CEOs of NBC and PSEG, elected officials, politicians, and other corporate executives. He currently works at a medical supply company in internal communications. Paul has a political science degree from Dickinson College and a Master's in Public Policy from the Kennedy School of Government, Harvard. He is an electric car enthusiast and speaker. Follow him on Twitter @PaulRosengren